AUTISM MOVEMENT THERAPY®
METHOD

WAKING UP THE BRAIN!

JOANNE LARA with Keri Bowers

Foreword by Stephen M. Shore

Jessica Kingsley *Publishers*
London and Philadelphia

First published in 2016
by Jessica Kingsley Publishers
73 Collier Street
London N1 9BE, UK
and
400 Market Street, Suite 400
Philadelphia, PA 19106, USA

www.jkp.com

Library of Congress Cataloging in Publication Data
Lara, Joanne, author.
  Autism movement therapy method : waking up the brain! / Joanne Lara with Keri Bowers ; foreword by Stephen M. Shore.
      p. ; cm.
The registered trademark symbol appears after the word therapy in the title.
Includes bibliographical references and index.
ISBN 978-1-84905-728-8 (alk. paper)
 I. Bowers, Keri, author. II. Title.
[DNLM: 1. Autistic Disorder--therapy. 2. Dance Therapy--methods. WS 350.8.P4]
RC489.D3
616.89'1655--dc23
                         2015017496

British Library Cataloguing in Publication Data
A CIP catalogue record for this book is available from the British Library

ISBN 978 1 84905 728 8
eISBN 978 1 78450 173 0

Printed and bound in Great Britain

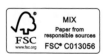

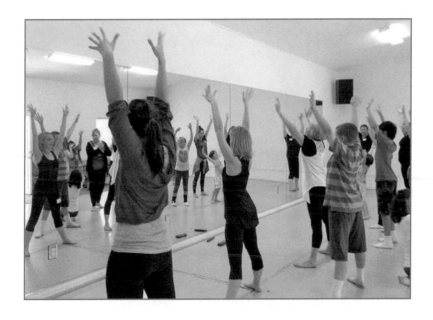

"Programs like Joanne's Autism Movement Therapy® offer opportunities for our kids to develop the necessary and fundamental skills that benefit all our kids. Art saved my life!"

TEMPLE GRANDIN, PHD

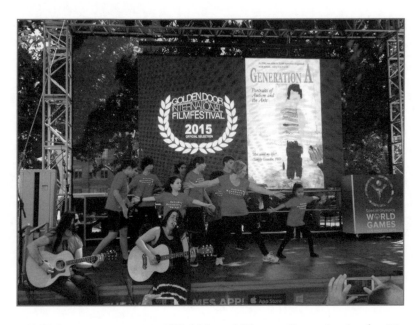

AMT dancers onstage at 2015 World Special Olympics Games, Los Angeles, CA

Contents

Foreword

Wake up! We all sense that chasing away sleepiness can be done with movement. For example, when traveling to distant countries, I know the most important thing for getting used to the new time zone is to move—especially when I can get out into the sunlight. Nothing gets a person going like moving to music. Even the March King, John Philips Sousa, said, "A good march should make a man with a wooden leg step out."

As a person on the autism spectrum I have intimate experience of the importance of music and movement. Regarding music, whatever it is that seems to scramble the speech and communication centers of the brain in people with autism and related conditions appears to leave the musical ones intact. Music therapists are aware of this as they strive to make human connections to those with autism and other conditions in the areas of communication, social interaction, motor control, and so on. I have seen great strides in interconnectedness in the students on the autism spectrum I give music lessons to.

Dr. Arnold Miller, co-developer of the Miller Method with his wife Eileen Eller-Miller, described difficulties individuals with autism have in differentiating between where their body ends and the environment begins. However, movement can be the best way to begin to make this differentiation. For example, while most people take for granted that they can reach behind them to touch the back of a chair they are sitting in, many on the autism spectrum lacking this important proprioceptive sense may, have to turn around and visually locate this part of the chair before touching it. Milder cases of difficulty in body-to-environmental awareness can be seen in clumsy individuals, who are often referred to as being like a "bull in a china shop," or not knowing their own strength.

Basing her work on the science of neurology and how the brain functions, Joanne Lara combines music and movement, creating a fun to implement intervention that is more powerful than the two parts alone. Perhaps my mother was aware of the power of combining music and movement, as a significant part of her, what we today refer to as "early intervention," consisted of some of the very things done in Autism Movement Therapy®.

A vital key to the success of Autism Movement Therapy is that it is *fun*! Wrapping sensory integration procedures, structured movement, music, modeling, and Positive Behavior Support, individuals engaging in the movements making up AMT train their brains to develop greater awareness and control of their bodies within their environment. This greater body efficacy overflows into improving communication, social interaction, self-esteem, and other areas of concern for people on the autism spectrum.

In additional to being a "must read," Autism Movement Therapy as described in *Austim Movement Therapy® Method: Waking up the brain,* by Joanne Lara with Keri Bowers, is a "must *experience*" for anyone wishing to learn how to empower individuals on the autism spectrum they support to first, be more comfortable within their bodies, and second, achieve greater success interacting with the surrounding environment. Having Autism Movement Therapy during my early days of being a significantly affected child on the autism spectrum would have been a great help. Fortunately, I had parents who intuitively understood what Joanne Lara and Keri Bowers have so expertly assembled in this book.

Stephen M. Shore, EdD
Clinical Assistant Professor at Adelphi University,
Internationally known author, speaker, and
individual on the autism spectrum

Acknowledgments

An enormous thank you from Keri Bowers and myself goes out to every person across the globe—in Europe, Asia, North America, South America, Africa, the Middle East and Australia—who are teaching our kiddos with autism and related disorders through the expressive arts. A special thank you to the over 600 Autism Movement Therapy® Certified providers and licensees who bring the 45 minute structured movement and music class to school rooms, auditoriums, dance studios, offices, community centers, government funded day programs and private homes to kids and youth across the globe. Whether it be music, movement, theater or the visual arts, what we know is that our students make incomparable progress when they have access to a structured art program. We are grateful to our friend and mentor, Dr. Temple Grandin, who reminds us that the arts require problem-solving skills, and when the brain and the body are asked to jump up and meet the bar and the bar is continually being raised, higher-level thinking skills must come into play. The brain and the body have to truly work as one unit, and it is through this combined brain and body effort that we—all of us—move from basic fundamental processing of the daily variables in our environment to deductive, inductive and finally analytical thinking processes.

I remain beholden to Chase Robinson, my University of South Florida dance faculty and Merce Cunningham dancer, who taught me while I was earning my Bachelor's in dance, that mediocre, whether in dance or in life, was just not good enough. I'm thankful to the late Louis Falco, who still remains a guide for me along with the late Billy Gornel, for allowing me to prove, to myself, that I wasn't a mediocre dancer or person. I am indebted to my colleague Alan Sener who remains a true friend to this day, though 38 years have passed since we, both light of mind and body, spent countless hours of sweat, hard work and joyful bliss on the sixth floor Falco Dance Studio loft on 24th street between 6th and 7th Avenues in New York City.

Autism Movement Therapy would not have been a reality without my mentors, Dr. Richard Mesaros, Dr. Ivor Weiner and the late Dr. June Downing from California State University Northridge (CSUN) in Los Angeles. Having spent six long years at CSUN earning my Moderate/Severe Education Specialist K–12 California Teaching Credential along with my Master's in Special Education: Moderate/Severe and Multiple Disabilities, while remaining a fully contracted special education teacher in Los Angeles Unified School District, I can honestly attribute all of my learned special education autism classroom teaching skills to these three fine educators. A heartfelt thank you also to Dr. KayDee Caywood, who continues to believe in me and my skills as a special educator by being my lead, my friend and a mentor at National University.

I am forever grateful to Paula Bennett, the assistant principal who gave me my first 3–5th grade autism special day classroom job in the Los Angeles Unified School District, where I was able to conceptualize and begin to develop the ideas of how important daily movement and music intervention were for our students with autism. I witnessed students who went from rolling on the floor and stimming on the overhead lights, to sitting at a computer, to assisting in a general education classroom, and ultimately to speaking, all through the power of music and movement.

I will be forever appreciative to my colleague, my friend, a remarkably talented visual artist and a warrior of a mother in the field of autism, who in 2007 sought me out at an autism conference in Pasadena, California and befriended me. Keri Bowers believed through first-hand experience, unlike the majority at that time, that the power of the arts could truly transform individuals and families. She understood without explanation that Autism Movement Therapy belonged at the table as an intervention for individuals with autism and related disorders, not just as a side bar, but as a daily intervention therapy to help the body and the mind perform as one unit, so that our students, our children and our friends could be the best that they could be.

And finally, I want to thank all my students over the course of those ten years in the public school setting, and my students today who are my teachers, who inspire me to get up every morning and try harder than the day before, to help show the world the potential that I know lives within each and every one of these remarkable human beings. I am truly blessed and continue to love my work, the students and the families that touch me daily. Namaste.

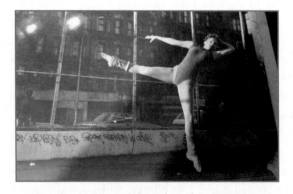

Joanne Lara, Amsterdam and 83rd St. NYC, 1980

Preface

"I observed here today what I should have had available to me in
my autism special needs school from 1953–1961. If I had the arts,
movement and music, I think I would be much further along than
I am now. Dance is good for everyone, regardless of age, autism or
neurology. I know that Autism Movement Therapy will enable me
to 'function better'."

LOUISE KAVADLO 2014

Louise arrived early on the second day of the Autism Movement Therapy®
(AMT) Certification workshop I was facilitating at the 92nd Street Y in
New York City. I had been asked before the start of the workshop by one
of the registered participants if her 67-year-old autistic sister might also
attend the two-day event. I agreed and welcomed Louise to attend the
second day of the ten-hour training.

After filling out her name tag, but before we started, Louise stayed close
by my side like sticky glue. After noticing her nervously follow me to the
restroom, I sensed her angst. AMT workshops are meant to engage and
relax participants—yet Louise was anything but relaxed. Trying to make
her more comfortable, I asked if she would like to stand closer to me at
the front of the class facing the mirrors when the class began. I smiled and
reassured Louise that she would do just fine.

To be clear, AMT is not "the wheels on the bus go round and round."
It's a 45-minute, formal, structured movement and music method that
stimulates the brain to "wake up" through audio, visual, gross motor
and imitation processing skills. Unlike my AMT class where students
imitate patterns and sequences in a structured, formatted dance class,

the certification workshop incorporates the 45-minute AMT class, and is designed for would-be trainers to learn the AMT processes and functions.

During the class, Louise struggled to get her brain to do what she wanted it to do, yet she worked diligently to follow along and participate. The emotions in the room were palpable. Tears welled up in everyone's eyes near the end of the class as an audible roar of applause from each of the 27 participants, myself included, cheered for Louise and her hard work. In all of her 67 years, Louise had never before experienced such freedom of her body's movement or the accomplishment of her brain's integration with the music and dance. With good reason, she was proud of her efforts and the outcome.

After viewing *Generation A: Portraits of Autism and the Arts*, a documentary I produced about five gifted individuals on the autism spectrum who excel in the arts, Louise raised her hand and said:

> I observed here today what I should have had available to me in my autism special needs school from 1953–1961. If I had the arts, movement and music, I think I would be much further along than I am now. Dance is good for everyone, regardless of age, autism or neurology. I know that Autism Movement Therapy will enable me to "function better." (Louise 2014)

Her words—the words of a true veteran warrior in autism—shot through me like a cannon ball. I've always wondered how things might be different if individuals with autism were encouraged to participate in the arts as a part of their everyday program of intervention. As Louise was sharing her experience, it came home to me that I was doing exactly what I had set out to do in 2007 when I created the foundation and processes for AMT.

I cannot imagine a world 20 years down the road where another individual like Louise tells us that the outcomes of who and what they had become as individuals would have been very different if they had had the opportunity to gain access to the arts.

This book is for all the Louises out there who are still fighting the good fight. Those who continue to advocate, grow and give back to their autism communities around the world. This book is for all of us who see the need—and desperately wish to fill it. This is for the lay person and the professional, and for the mindful beauty of the arts and autism.

Joanne Lara, MA Certified Core Adjunct Faculty,
National University, College of Education, Department of
Special Education Founder Autism Movement Therapy, Inc

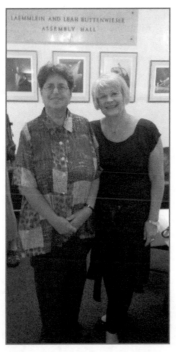

Louise Kavadlo and Joanne Lara, 92nd St Y Harkness Dance Center, 2014

PART I

UNDERSTANDING AUTISM MOVEMENT THERAPY®

CHAPTER 1

The Benefits of a Movement and Music Program

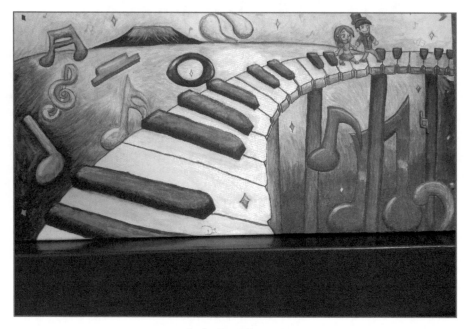

Art by Dani Bowman

"When we move we coordinate our brain. Autism Movement Therapy® helped me coordinate my body too. When I was younger, I thought it would just be free dance, but I like that we have a routine basically."

EMMA ELIZABETH BATHUM, 14 YEARS OLD

Movement and music makes a profound impact on individuals with autism. One of the most exciting discoveries we've made in the 40 plus years of our individual and collective work in autism is how art expression, including movement and dance, profoundly impacts people with autism. Young and old, boys and girls, men and women, verbal and non-verbal—we've watched how participation in the arts improves and builds essential skills in many areas of autism's core deficits of speech and language, social skills and behavioral challenges.

The expressive arts give rise to communication for the voiceless, meaning to the intangible and comprehension to the mysteries of human interactions. Participation in movement and music provides a literal and metaphoric stage upon which to share the inner being of our souls. Yet movement and music gives opportunities for much more. As the economy dwindles, and the demand for intensive, viable therapies in autism rises, the need for affordable—low cost or free—interventions became imperative. Can you imagine a simple, accessible program in movement and music that could meet many of those needs? Can you imagine having fun while growing and learning in autism?

Science is finally beginning to study the effects of the expressive arts on autism—and it's about time. Steven Kapp, an autism researcher at the University of California, Los Angeles tells us, "Now that the autism field has begun to intensively study sensory-movement differences, they have become better understood, with potential to spur change" (Kapp 2013). Research is beginning to support what we've discovered through Autism Movement Therapy (AMT) and other art forms for decades; that an early intervention program that includes the expressive arts is fundamentally productive and the outcomes can (and do) drastically benefit the child's needs. The arts provide powerful, results-based strategies for autistic individuals through solid, well-conceived and structured programs such as AMT that literally *wake up the brain*! We invite you to come along with us on this journey of exploration and possibilities to see for yourself the rewards in store for you, your child, your students and your clients.

MOVEMENT AND MUSIC HELPS DEVELOP ESSENTIAL CORE SKILLS

In addition to simple, fun exercise and social interaction, AMT helps to develop essential skills and positively affects autism's challenges, including:

- speech, language and communication

- gross and fine motor skills/planning

- proprioception, balance and spatial orientation

- sensory processing and integration

- social and life skills

- physical health and wellness

- self-esteem, self-awareness and self-determination

- anxiety and depression.

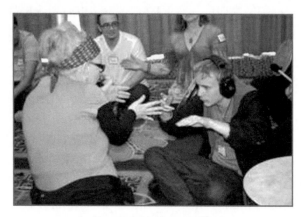

Keri with Neal AMT class

With hundreds of anecdotal, real-life stories of how AMT has benefited the autistic kids and adults we've worked with, it's a simple brush stroke to share how, for example, 20-year-old student, Neal, willingly relinquished his headphones to "tolerate" the music and boisterous interactions of an afternoon session at a week-long AMT spring class. The immediate benefits to Neal were apparent. Neal's sensory integration issues (sound), social and spatial awareness (proximity to others in a group), and communication skills (improved ability to convey his needs during our sessions) increased. The pleasurable and fluid nature of AMT movement and music, by its nature, puts kids at ease, relaxing their minds and bodies. Neal is one example of this. We will reveal why this occurs in coming chapters.

"Joanne's class helped make my balance better. I feel good about that."

EMMA, AGED 13

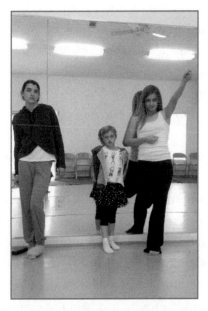

Emma, aged 10, is in the center

It is typical for children like Emma to start out in AMT classes with behavioral challenges, anxiety and body balance/coordination deficits. At eight years old, Emma was unsure—or unaware—of where her body was situated in relationship to the environment and people around her (poor body-to-environment challenge). In class, she was significantly challenged by the movements and routines of AMT. Carol Kranowitz tells us in her book *The Out-of-Sync Child* that oftentimes perceptual motor therapy, or integrated movement experiences that remediate gross-motor, fine-motor and visual discrimination problems, stimulate alternative routes to the memory and sequencing for children who do not respond to the methods taught in the conventional classroom (2005, p.224).

For years, Emma had participated in intensive occupational therapy (OT). OT had helped with many of her challenges, but in this new environment, Emma was unable to move her body as a unit through space in the class. Whether attempting to imitate the instructions of "arms in the air," "feet apart," "feet together," or just execute simple slides across the room, Emma struggled to move her body parts in unison. Her head, like many kids with autism, preceded her body as she crossed the floor, her legs behind her. Her brain was not wired (yet) to send the proper and necessary signals to her body for her to follow the routines. *Note: We say "yet," because the very idea of changing or altering brain connectivity after a certain age remains controversial amongst experts. But we believe in the concept of neuroplasticity, as we will discuss in Chapter 2, which supports the idea that the brain can indeed form new connections that improve both physical and mental abilities.*

The initial expectations for Emma when she began taking the AMT class in the winter of 2008 were two-fold: a) to help her to become comfortable in the environment; and b) to introduce her to the AMT movement patterns and sequences. She also needed time to adjust to yet another new and unfamiliar teacher in her life. After several weeks, and as Emma's trust in the environment grew, she began to bond with her class peers and become more comfortable in her new surroundings. It was exciting to see whole body movements begin to emerge. Over time, Emma developed more confidence and enjoyment in the sessions. She did not become comfortable with becoming a leader for at least a year…but with us wanting all kids to be leaders, it happened. Not all children are ready in the beginning, but all of them flourish when they become leader. They let us know when they are ready.

SAY "CHEESE!"

Looking at old film footage of Emma is one way we can see her improvement over time. It is useful to use video and film to document dance, drama, music and art sessions; that way, you can create a realistic visual and auditory baseline of the child's present level of performance, and then, over time, you and the parents can document growth and development just like you would in a classroom setting. The parents appreciate this as well. "Seeing" is generally better than "telling," and "asking" always trumps telling. When we ask, we stimulate the higher-level thinking skills thereby "waking up the brain." Case in point, if you "tell your student to go put his backpack away in the cubby," you have not required the brain to do any "work," but if you ask, "where do you need to put your backpack?" then you have asked the brain to engage. To formulate a question requires a thought process for an answer. This very act of the student thinking "where *do* I need to put my backpack?" activates lobes in the brain and stimulates neurons.

Videotaping a child is also a highly useful and effective tool to use in helping a child to "see" themselves. When they see how they present themselves to the world; what their body, their movements and facial expressions look like, new discussions and learning can unfold. Keri used to film and photograph her son, Taylor, when he was a young boy. Taylor is now 27 years old and lives independently through state and federal funding in a small town in southern California. From the time he was one year old and couldn't crawl or talk, Keri would show him video footage or photographs and ask: "What does Taylor see?" or "Is Taylor happy or sad?" Because he could not speak outside of unintelligible babbles—it would be years before he would speak—she would talk to him as if he understood her. Keri's intuition and her heart told her he would understand her words if she acted as if he could. This is what we mean by raising the bar.

Keri would add opinions to her questions such as, "It looks to me like Taylor feels sad. Is Taylor sad?" Then she would frown to help model the expression of "sad." Over time, in the years and language that ultimately followed, Taylor emerged as reasonably sensitive to the emotions and feelings of self and others. He was self-aware, and able to look outside of his previously isolated world. Was this an accident or simply normal development? Considering autism, I don't think so. It was hard work, creativity and dedication that brought this inward, isolated child out into the light.

THE EASE AND NATURALLY ENJOYABLE ASPECTS OF AUTISM MOVEMENT THERAPY

Whether verbal or non-verbal, students new to AMT methods often start the classes overwhelmed and overstimulated. Kids who are bombarded by a barrage of daily and/or weekly therapies are often emotionally and physically oversaturated by interventions beyond school-time activities. Though highly valuable, Applied Behavior Analysis (ABA), speech and language, OT and other more rigid interventions overload our children. That is partly why the organically fun nature of AMT can be a welcome relief over traditional therapies. Of course there are structure and expectations that students must follow, but those expectations are "hidden" within the framework of this more relaxed, "recreational" activity. In more intense interventions, obedience determines the reward. In AMT, just being a part of the expressive movement and music is the reward—and the skills gained are the benefits.

The ease and naturally enjoyable aspects of movement and music are key factors in seeing a group of kids—who start out as Neal and Emma did with core anxiety and behavioral issues—transform, flourish and eagerly perform in sync with one another. When our core AMT group in Los Angeles performs in live stage productions, it is a brilliant phenomenon to witness the bright faces and fierce determination of the participants to perform their roles. When the stage lights go on, the curtains go up and the show begins, tears begin flowing from family members; moms and dads who were initially leery that *their child* could actually perform live on a stage. This happens every time! We make contingencies for those kids who might elope or get stage fright, but we never have to use those contingencies because the reward is in the movement and music, and kids are inspired to "show up" for the show.

SHOSHANA'S JOURNEY

The earlier snapshots shared of both Neal and Emma are preludes to the more in-depth case study of Shoshana. Her story will surely inspire a vivid picture of a typical AMT student from the first early sessions to the present day. We will also share some of Shoshana's personal experiences of AMT's effects on her life, and include her mother's perspective on her daughter's growth and development over the years as well.

As you read this book and get to know more about the AMT method and Shoshana, we ask you to consider how her story and the results she has experienced might feel to you. What if your own child, student or client were able to achieve similar results? How might life change for your child if his or her core skills improved? How might your life experiences be different? How might autism's challenges be reframed? *Autism Movement Therapy® Method: Waking up the Brain!* will show you how you can bring this easily adaptable method into your home, school or organization.

WHAT IS AUTISM MOVEMENT THERAPY?

When I left my credentialed teaching position in the Los Angeles Unified School District classroom, where I had taught students with moderate/severe disabilities for over ten years in a special day class setting, and where I first began incorporating music and movement into the daily classroom schedule, I suspected but did not entirely understand the profound role that music and movement would play in actual speech and language production. It was that teaching experience and the ability to work with hundreds of kids in those early years that lent itself to the development and goals of the AMT method.

AMT is a fun, empowering sensory integration tool. The AMT method blends multi-sensory, structured movement and music experiences with Positive Behavior Support (PBS) to connect the left and right hemispheres of the brain. AMT appeals to all people of all ages, and supports strengthening and building a "whole brain," cognitive approach—or interhemispheric integration—to significantly increase skills and behaviors through the body and brain connection.

AMT combines patterning, visual movement calculation, audile[1] receptive processing, rhythm and sequencing into "whole brain" cognitive thinking skills through connections that can significantly impact and improve a wide variety of autism's deficits. AMT is a natural strategy for individuals with autism and related disorders, and provides individuals with limited speech and language communication skills in particular,

---

1   A person whose mental imagery consists of sounds (Merriam-Webster Medical Dictionary).

a way to express what words fail to do. AMT allows the non-verbal or impaired verbal individual self-expression through music and movement while developing a strong sense of self-determination and independence, undoubtedly one of the most important tools that the student will develop in their skill set.

BIG DREAMS, BIG GOALS

The primary goal of AMT is that after 12–14 weeks of two or three 12-minute sessions per week (as demonstrated in the AMT *aut-erobics* DVD[2]), or one 45-minute AMT class over the same time period, the individual will be more compliant when asked to complete on-task activities, will interact with typical general education peers more frequently and will have better use of the four lobes of the brain for processing. Increased overall self-determination awareness and self-regulation, along with healthier, improved self-esteem that equates to community inclusion and job opportunities is the ultimate goal. We always ask parents where they see their child in 5, 10, 15 years. As parents, this can be a frightening question to ponder. AMT offers a way to track progress and encourage the development of skills that will be necessary to support inclusive futures. With big dreams and big goals, the AMT method helps us to see those possibilities.

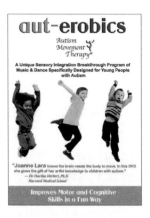

Aut-erobics DVD cover

---

2   The *aut-erobics (Autism Movement Therapy)* DVD can be purchased on the Autism Movement Therapy website at www.autismmovementtheraphy.org, along with the documentary that features the Autism Movement Therapy method, *Generation A: Portraits of Autism and the Arts*, with Dr. Temple Grandin and Dr. Stephen Shore. AMT Certification workshop information is also available.

"When I moved, my body felt free. Being so tall and not in shape I felt exhausted. The upside of feeling exhausted, like going to the gym, is walking away feeling more alert. AMT did that for me."

TAYLOR CROSS, 22, AUTISM; CO-CREATOR,
NORMAL PEOPLE SCARE ME

The wonderful news about AMT is that while we typically need to intervene early with traditional therapies, studies indicate that sensory integration therapies can be effective with autistic individuals past the toddler stage, offering new hope to older children and even adults (Woo and Leon 2013).

BRAIN MATTER: WHAT THE HECK IS NEUROPLASTICITY?

The premise and underlying foundation of *Autism Movement Therapy®Method: Waking up the Brain!* begins with the brain, which is a vastly complex and baffling organ.

Despite its mysteries, our brain has an amazing natural capacity to compensate for injury or disease throughout our life. The ability to reorganize and form new connections, synapses (chemical or electrical connection points between brain cells), or create neural pathways in our nervous system is called "neuroplasticity." Though controversial, the science of neuroplasticity is based on the idea that the adult brain is capable of improving cognition and/or restoring lost mental abilities and function through regular, continuous physical and mental activities.

While scientists once believed the brain was a static (fixed or unchangeable) organ, research is changing that position by exploring how—and in which ways—the brain changes throughout life. In *The Brain That Changes Itself*, author Norman Doidge illuminates case histories and research that indicate that the brain is far more malleable than we once thought (Doidge 2007). His work supports the idea that learning a new skill actually changes the structure and function of the brain—even into old age. Together and individually, our anecdotal experience with AMT and other programs in the arts agrees with this view. We have seen first-hand, literally hundreds of children over two decades restore lost or underdeveloped skills well into their teens and adulthood.

It is because of the successes we have witnessed with our own eyes that we have developed a firm respect and belief in the science of neuroplasticity. With that in mind, the AMT method shows how the use of repetitive patterns and sequencing via movement and music literally wakes up the parts of the brain in individuals with autism—and related disorders—that are dormant or not receiving neural stimulation.

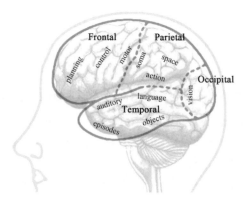

The four lobes of the brain

OUR BRAINS ARE LIKE COMPUTERS

Like a computer, our brain is an information-processing wonder. This mysterious wonder retrieves, decodes, processes and stores information in either long-term or short-term areas of our brain. When we need a particular piece or pieces of information, we retrieve it via a pathway called "white brain matter" in the mapping area (gray matter) of the brain.

So how do our brains process the "variables" in our environment? What exactly is the "job" of each of the four lobes in our brain? And how do sensory enrichment therapies increase cognitive abilities while at the same time decrease common autistic behaviors? Brain mapping is beginning to give us these answers.

Brain mapping is an interesting and complex process. Scientists have used imaging to map and watch the brain working on various tasks. While this complex super-computer remains in large part a mystery, research is making great strides in better understanding how the brain works. We know that there is a part of the brain whose function is vision, and another whose function is primarily sound. Brain mapping is helping us to look deeper into the vision section to see if there is differentiation within the brain that is responsible, say, for detecting a certain area, the color red, or another area detecting the color green, or the same area detecting both red and green? Brain mapping, or cognitive redirection as it is also known, looks from the outside in and seeks to understand how the environment affects the brain and how in turn the brain changes because of environmental stimuli.

In a nutshell, it's like this: Say you move into a new home in a new neighborhood. You don't know where to find the grocery store, the dry cleaner, your bank or any other neighborhood establishments you need on a daily basis. But soon, after you've located these places, you no longer have to think about the specific directions to get to any of them. Your brain has "mapped" these locations, so you are able to get into your car and drive right to the spot, almost as though you're on "automatic pilot." Every day we map hundreds of pieces of information by placing them in a file in our brain. Without even having to think about it, when we need certain information we retrieve the file by going straight to it, via cognitive maps or highway pathways.

Individuals with autism have difficulty accessing and retrieving information in both long- and/or short-term memory banks. Either the pathway does not exist or the transmitters are impaired. In either case, the cognitive maps are not working efficiently, if at all. This makes learning especially difficult. The analogy is that the person's brain functions like a library where none of the information is stored in any organized, categorized way. Think of the confusion this would cause! The good news is that scientists now know we can often jumpstart impaired informational pathways or even create new pathways through cognitive redirection or, as discussed earlier, neuroplasticity (Lara 2009).

THE CORPUS CALLOSUM: UNDERSTANDING THE LEFT AND RIGHT BRAIN HEMISPHERES

The corpus callosum is a thick band of nerve fibers that divides the brain into the left and right hemispheres. The job of the corpus callosum is to transfer motor, sensory and cognitive information between the left and right brain areas. This communication helps maintain balance, regulate eye movement, uphold an equilibrium between arousal and attention, and to assist with tactile discrimination from the outside environment.

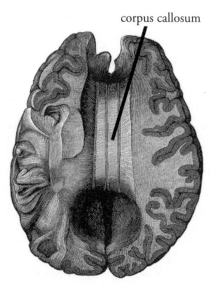

Brain showing the corpus callosum

In a typical brain, information from the environment is received and travels across the corpus callosum, which is much like a bridge, supporting this communication. For many individuals with autism, however, the left and right brain hemispheres have difficulty communicating with each other. Research points to the fact that kids with autism have a smaller corpus callosum and studies seem to indicate that this inability of the left and right hemispheres to communicate is one of the underlying core challenges for individuals with autism (Frazier *et al.* 2012).

Einstein had an extremely thick corpus callosum. According to a study in 2013 by Men *et al.* published in the journal *Brain*, Einstein's corpus callosum at the time of his death was thicker in the vast majority of subregions than the corporas callosa of 15 elderly healthy males, and thicker at five key crossings than those of 52 young, healthy males who served as a comparison group (Men *et al.* 2013).

In most neurotypical (NT) people either the left or the right hemisphere is dominant at any given time, but in individuals with autism one side of the brain tends to always be more dominant than the other.

The left (analytic) or logical hemisphere of the brain is:

- verbal

- responds to word meaning

- is sequential

- processes information linearly

- responds to logic and plans ahead

- recalls people's names

- speaks with few gestures

- is punctual

- prefers formal study design

- prefers bright lights while studying.

The right (global) or artistic hemisphere is:

- visual

- responds to tone of voice

- is random and processes information in varied order

- responds to emotion

- is impulsive

- recalls people's faces

- gestures when speaking

- is less punctual

- prefers sound or music in the background while studying and prefers frequent mobility while studying.

In order for the brain to function as a "whole brain," the left and right hemispheres must be exchanging information/talking with one another.

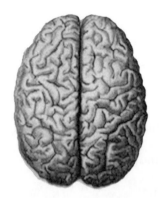

The brain's left and right hemispheres

THE CEREBRAL CORTEX: INFORMATION HIGHWAY

Information in our environment is received via the cerebral cortex, which is a vital layer of tissue that coats the surface of the brain, with roughly the thickness of two or three dimes stacked. The word "cortex" comes from the Latin word for tree bark—perhaps so named for its wrinkly appearance. The cortex is a huge communication system, playing a key role in basic functions such as memory, attention, perceptual awareness, planning movements, and making sense of information from our eyes and ears. It is also responsible for more advanced functions such as language and abstract thought.

cerebral cortex

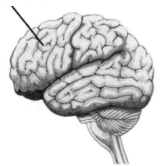

CEREBRAL CORTEX: A huge communication system, which plays a key role in memory, attention, perceptual awareness, planning movements and making sense of information from our eyes and ears. It is also responsible for advanced functions such as language and abstract thought.

The cerebral cortex

Variations in the structure of the cortex might explain why an NT person and an autistic person who receive the same sensory information interpret or experience the information in completely different ways. Whether you are a parent or a professional, surely you will find the following "mis-association" interpretation example familiar. A child with autism goes to the park with his father. He sees a dog and leans down to pet it. Simultaneously, his father looks up at the sky and says, "What a lovely blue sky." A month later, the boy sees a dog at a friend's home. He immediately rushes over and as he lovingly pets the dog he says, "blue sky"—the words he cognitively mapped and stored in his memory bank during his trip to the park. The boy is re-experiencing the same activity, one that he enjoyed, so his brain retrieves the words (speech—frontal and parietal lobes) he heard from his father (receptive audio information—temporal lobe) that were stored along with the picture of the dog (visual—occipital lobe) and the action of petting the dog (gross motor—cerebellum). When the child says "blue sky," adults then misinterpret and misunderstand the child as thinking the name of the dog is "Blue Sky." In actual fact, the image of the dog was the visual trigger for the retrieval of the stored information in the boy's brain.

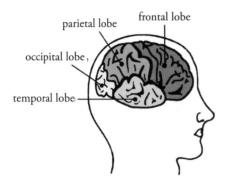

parietal lobe   frontal lobe

occipital lobe

temporal lobe

FRONTAL LOBE: Concerned with reasoning, planning, parts of speech and movement (motor cortex), emotions and problem-solving. Often referred to as the "Executive Functioning" area of the brain.

Brain showing the four lobes

Each of us processes information in this same manner. The difference between processing the correct information and/or misinformation, as in the above example, is dependent on the negative or positive interpretation of the information. We process through audio, visual and natural cues, which in turn become triggers. In other words, we can see something or hear it, or both see it and hear it together in order to establish a trigger. In the example of your cat meowing to let you know he wants to be fed, you can see the cat near his bowl, or you can hear the cat from another room, or you can see and hear the cat in order to trigger you to go to the cabinet and pull down a can of cat food. AMT utilizes these different forms of information processing and triggers in remapping the brain. It requires the individual to use receptive language to hear the music, visual processing to see the physical image and gross motor skills to reproduce what they see.

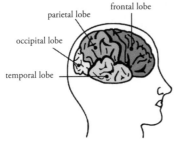

TEMPORAL LOBE: Concerned with perception and recognition of auditory stimuli (hearing) and memory (hippocampus).

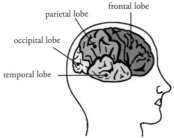

PARIETAL LOBE: Concerned with perception of stimuli related to touch, pressure, temperature and pain.

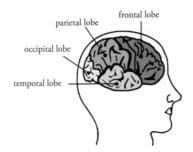

OCCIPITAL LOBE: Located at the back of the brain, behind the parietal lobe and temporal lobe. Concerned with aspects of vision.

Brain showing the four lobes

The wonderful news about AMT is that the method offers new hope to parents of older children and even adults. While we typically intervene with traditional therapies such as OT, ABA and speech and language as soon as a child receives an autism diagnosis, studies indicate that sensory integration therapies can also be effective with individuals who are past the toddler stage (Woo and Leon 2013). AMT is based on the concept of neuroplasticity, the belief that the brain, rather than being fixed, can change. Change brought about through a movement and music program often has a profound effect on the speech and language processing areas of the brain. We have seen tremendous progress in the Wernicke's area of the brain, located at the posterior end of the temporal lobe that is responsible for the pragmatics of ideas of language, as well as the Broca area, which lives in the frontal lobe and controls speech articulation. Both the Broca and the Wernicke's reside in the left hemisphere of the brain.

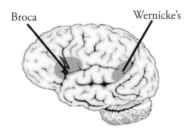

Brain Broca and Wernicke's

SHOSHANA'S FIRST AMT CLASS

Shoshana attended her first AMT class in 2008. She was eight years old, had a limited attention span and a very limited communication system. She had a Picture Exchange Communication System (PECS) to communicate with others, but preferred throwing herself on the floor, screaming at a high pitch and running full speed into the dance studio walls. All, for the most part, sensory seeking behaviors.

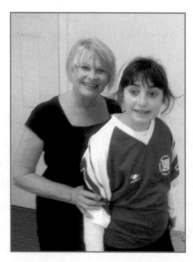

Shoshana and Joanne in an AMT class (2008)

EVIDENCE OF SUCCESS

More and more, researchers are collecting data that supports empirical evidence of the very real therapeutic values of music and movement in autism. In 2001 at the University of Miami School of Medicine, Kristin Hartshorn and her team conducted a study on 38 children with autism who were given movement therapy in small groups led by a trained movement therapist. After two months of bi-weekly sessions, the children spent less time wandering, more time showing on-task behavior, less time showing negative responses to being touched, and less time resisting the teacher than those in the control group (Hartshorn *et al.* 2001).

In 2013, a study performed at University of California (UC), Irvine, comprised of two groups of children with autism, revealed stunning results. The control group consisted of 15 children with autism, ranging in age from 3–12 years who were given standard conventional treatment for autism (ABA, OT, speech and Physical therapy); meanwhile, the study group, consisting of 13 children, also ranging in age from 3–12 years, were given a variety of sensory enrichment therapies. In a six-month period of time, the authors reported a five point increase on the Childhood Autism Rating Scale™ (CARS™) as well as an IQ increase of ten points (Woo and Leon 2013) in the sensory enrichment group. These are not only significant findings, they are profound.

CARS is a diagnostic assessment method that rates children on a scale from one to four for various criteria, ranging from normal to severe, and then yields a composite score ranging from non-autistic to mildly autistic, moderately autistic, or severely autistic. The scale is used to observe and subjectively rate 15 items: relationship to people, imitation, emotional response, body, object use, adaptation to change, visual response, listening response, taste/smell/touch response, fear and nervousness, verbal communication, non-verbal communication, activity level, level and consistency of intellectual response and general impressions (Schopler *et al.* 1980). A five-point increase on the CARS can literally move a child from autistic to non-autistic in one fell swoop.

As the UC Irvine study group reported, and as the AMT method has anecdotally demonstrated over and over again, the more information that travels across the corpus callosum—that wide, flat bundle of nerve fibers beneath the cortex—and the more access to stimulation in the left and right hemispheres, the more chance that visual, audio and gross motor processing growth can occur. The benefits, however, are not only seen in processing functions, but in the storing and retrieving of information in a more efficient and effective manner. How can this be possible?

Think of it like a laundry room. You buy a new home with a guest house in the back yard. No one has ever lived in the guest house, and the back yard grass is green, lovely and covers the entire ground. Your friend or relative moves into the guest house, and they use your laundry room, located at the back of your house. After a while, inevitably a pathway forms from the guest house to the laundry room. This is how we make new pathways in the brain, by having the information travel back and forth, over and over again, along the same white brain matter transmitters until the brain establishes that the traveled route is the preferred pathway to the stored information. Doesn't sound so impossible after all, right?

THE DALI LAMA, THE BRAIN AND MEDITATION

When the Dali Lama teamed up with Wall Street journalist and author of *Train Your Mind, Change Your Brain* (2007), Sharon Begley, to speak at the annual meeting of the Society for Neuroscience, the world's largest gathering of brain scientists, in 2005, the Dali Lama asked the attendees to ponder the following key idea:

> In addition to the brain giving rise to thoughts and hopes and beliefs and emotions that add up to this thing we call the mind, maybe the mind also acts back on the brain to cause physical changes in the very matter that created it. If so, then pure thought would change the brain's activity, its circuits or even its structure.

Sharon Begley, author of *Train Your Mind, Change Your Brain*, went on to say:

> Recent pioneering experiments in neuroplasticity, a new science that investigates whether and how the brain can undergo wholesale change, reveal that the brain is capable not only of altering its structure but also of generating new neurons, even into old age. The brain can adapt, heal, renew itself after trauma, and compensate for disability. (Begley 2007)

Following his lecture the Dali Lama later arranged for Tibetan monks to travel to American universities for magnetic resonance imaging (MRI) brain scans to measure the changes that meditation brought about in the brain. Imagine that…combining music and movement with meditation to heal the brain's neurological dysfunctions!

Notwithstanding the encouraging results of relatively limited research and longitudinal studies into autism, the arts, music and movement, currently we see that music therapy has the largest body of evidence to support its efficacy for students in special education—especially those with autism. Scientists hypothesize that music engages the mirror neuron system in the human brain, which supports development in sensory-motor integration, speech and social skills (McGarry and Russo 2011; Wang 2014).The AMT method simply adds movement to the science of music "therapy" to increase the developmental and educational benefits to those engaging in the processes.

We encourage—and one day fully expect to see—evidence-based research on the arts, substantially qualifying them as viable, scientific interventions in autism. And one day, we envision the arts will become "Best Practices" in autism therapies. These Best Practices would incorporate along with speech and language, audio, visual and gross motor processing growth, a strong imitation, visualization and pairing of speech and language. AMT, like ABA, utilizes a solid imitation component along with a visualization development piece that is built into the final portion of the class where the students slowly lie down on the ground, roll flat on their back, close their eyes and think of their body melting into the floor. Then we visit "in our mind," say for example, the beach. I ask each student to imagine that they are on a beach, then I ask each student one by one to tell us what they see on the beach. Building a strong visualization association process in the brain requires re-mapping the cerebral cortex, the communication system that we spoke about earlier, the bark that covers the brain and transmits information to its four lobes. Imitation requires abstract thought, so rather than the familiar concrete thinking that comes more naturally to our kids with autism, we must scaffold the visualization process and build, if you will, the ability for our kids to visualize or experience imagination. Imagination is one of the first questions asked of the parent on the Autism

Diagnostic Interview™—Revised (ADI™-R) (Rutter *et al.* 2005), one of the two fundamental universal autism assessment tools, the other being the Autism Diagnostic Observation Schedule™ (ADOS™) (Lord *et al.* 1989) used to establish eligibility of autism.

CHAPTER 2

What Does an Autism Movement Therapy® Session Look Like?

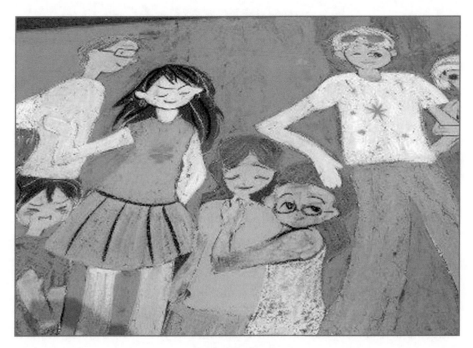

Art by Keri Bowers

"There's a bridge between the left and right hemisphere that transmits information. What happens with our kids is that the transmission of the information is not going through. Dance and music forces the brain to reorganize itself. Through the music and the movement the child is being asked to hear the music, process the sequence and the patterns, and then dance; it takes both sides of the brain to dance."

JOANNE LARA, 2010

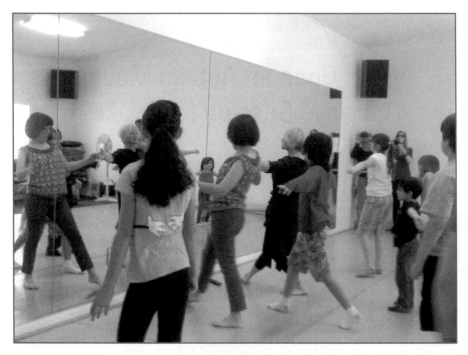

AMT class

INCLUSION WITH NEUROTYPICAL PEERS
AND AUTISM MOVEMENT THERAPY

On any given Saturday morning in the quiet suburbs of Los Angeles, 15–20 kids gather to participate in a one-hour, ongoing AMT class. AMT is delivered in Los Angeles in a full inclusion setting, meaning there are NT students as well as students with challenges in the class. Studies indicate that inclusive settings offer role model awareness and opportunities that cannot be replicated in a setting where there are only individuals with autism or related disabilities (Chan and O'Reilly 2008, p.405).

An inclusive setting allows for meaningful opportunities for increased social interaction. A core criteria deficit of individuals with autism and Asperger's is weak social skills. An inclusive setting, a mixed setting with NT as well as individuals with autism, offers increased opportunities for our students to see, imitate and model appropriate behavior, with the idea that the student will not only imitate but generalize this appropriate social behavior in other environmental settings such as home, school and community. Inclusion also creates additional oppurtunities for our students with autism to hear language used with the correct syntax (order and meaning) and in turn use these words in correct sentence structure with the desired intention (Ellis 1996).

Most importantly, our students with autism learn new skills and make friends with NT students, and the NT students learn how to be friends with kids with autism and disabilities, increasing the opportunity for jobs and community inclusion for our students after they transition out of the public school setting. A win-win for everyone!

So instead of transitioning to the back room of their parents' home with a DVD player after graduating, we can assist our individuals with autism in getting and keeping a job, possibly living independently or in a supported living center, having meaningful relationships with others and in becoming a productive member of their society and community at large. Employment for individuals with autism in the United States and globally is devastatingly low.

SHOSHANA AND SOCIAL LANGUAGE

Shoshana is often one of the first to arrive. After taking off her shoes, she paces around the room, eager to see who will show up for class. Over the years, Shoshana has emerged from her cocoon as an inward, isolated young girl, who once threw herself against the dance studio walls, to become a vibrant, chattering teenaged butterfly. She's become a diligent helper in the class, eagerly encouraging newcomers and all the others to participate in the routine activities of the day. Shoshana has become a leader in the group—confident and capable. And most important of all, Shoshana came to AMT with a very limited speech and language skill set—much of her antisocial behavior stemmed from her inability to communicate effectively with peers and adults in her environment. After five years in the Saturday AMT class, Shoshana is constructing 7–8 word sentences and is not only able to get her fundamental wants and needs met, but now uses language to communicate socially with peers and adults.

Shoshana's mother, Andrea, explains that since taking her daughter to AMT class for the past six years, she and her husband, Irv, have noticed the following changes and/or improvements:

- More compliance and willingness to follow directions.

- When she began the class, Shoshana was non-verbal; she now has functional speech and she is working on conversational speech.

- Shoshana's focus and eye contact have improved and continue to improve.

- Shoshana now has an understanding of "questions" and she is able to exhibit short-term recall.

- Shoshana is able to watch, process and imitate the movement and patterns in the AMT class.

- Shoshana considers the other children in the class as her friends and enjoys seeing them every week.

- From a personal point of view, Andrea and Irv feel that AMT has also helped Shoshana tremendously by teaching them how to work with their daughter to help her reach her greatest potential.

GETTING STARTED

With the music cued to begin with Eric Bibb's "Don't Ever Let Nobody Drag Your Spirit Down," the "Everybody on your dot," direct verbal prompt is given. We stand, arms stretched out to our sides and legs apart in second position, heads held high, facing the wall-length mirror to begin our usual warm-up. The single most important key to success in any movement and music class for children is that each student knows their "place" in the room or the environment. For this very reason, AMT embraces "the dot" concept. "The dot" concept or theory of knowing where to be in our environment carries over into all areas for our kids with autism. The importance of knowing one's place in the room, neighborhood, classroom and, ultimately, the world, cannot be stressed enough. Individuals with autism struggle with the challenge of processing all the variables in their surroundings. This includes stimuli such as sound, light and objects coming at them at the same time, bombarding them sensorily. Depending on the neurological design of the brain, which determines how the information in the enviornment is being received, identified and then processed by the brain, each child is different in the way that they will interpret the variables. We must use direct instruction and literally point to and maneuver the child to the painter's tape (see Box 2.1) on the floor, to show or indicate to the student where their position is in the dance room. Knowing one's position in any given environment—in the world if you will—for all of us, at any given moment, is fundamental to our immediate and future success and directly related to how we will react in any given moment. So, knowing where you stand in the AMT dance room is in direct proportion to how successful you will be in the class.

In the beginning, this is one of the toughest elements of AMT to teach: the student will often want to run in circles around the other students, or in and out of the students as they are standing on their dots waiting to begin the first warm-up song. This is natural, but what we want is to redirect the student back to their "dot" or position in the class. So the dot serves as a "home base," if you will—the place that the student will always come back to during the warm-up. Later in the class, we will also establish two additional rows of dots, spaced approximately 1.5 feet apart (45cm) on both sides of the room, which will act in the same manner, letting the student know where they belong in the room as they move/dance across the floor from side to side.

DOOR

PARENTS OR CARE GIVERS CAN SIT IN CHAIRS ACROSS THE BACK OF THE ROOM

```
+  +  +  + ++ + +  +        +  +  + +  +  + +  +  +

  X      X    X    X    X    X    X    X    X

    X    X    X    X    X    X    X    X    X

+  + + + + + + +         +  + + +  + + +  + +
```

TEACHER STANDS FACING THE MIRROR

■

Mirror

Key AMT classroom floor layout

■: Teacher

X: Student (dot—blue or colored painter's tape on floor)

+: Student line-up row dots for moving across
the floor from one side to the other

Figure of set up for classroom

BOX 2.1 STAYING ON TASK

In AMT sessions, we've established that our "best friend" will be the colored painter's tape. I use blue. Using colored tape or dots, although most colored dots have sticky glue on the back and oftentimes if you are teaching a class in a dance studio or a school auditorium the establishment doesn't take kindly to the residue that is left from the back of the dots on the floor, which is why painter's tape is really the best choice.

The markers should be placed approximately 3–4 feet (90–120cm) apart, in order to give the participants ample space between themselves and their peers during the ten-minute warm-up.

You will want to use tape on the floor even if you are working with only one child—for example, in your living room, office or classroom—to help them regulate over time where they start and stop, which will eventually help to establish the idea of where their place is in space and in the world. The visual cue (the tape) will later be the trigger to "where do I belong in this room, in this space, in this environment?"

RAISING THE BAR OF EXPECTATIONS

I would say that our kids typically live in a world of confusion, anxiety and stress. Depending on the degree of cognitive impairment, many times nothing in their environment makes any sense. If they have receptive processing deficits, then the language that they are hearing doesn't mean anything to them and different sound frequencies may be dropping in and out. Couple this with expressive language processing impairment—they are not able to speak or tell us what they don't know—along with visual processing impairment, and it is no wonder many children with autism elope, running out of rooms, down hallways and into streets. We would most likely react the same way if people in our environment continued to speak to us in loud tones, close to our face, and for hours on end. It is our job as parents, teachers, caregivers and service providers to help make their world as simple and clear as we can for then so that they can function to the best of their abilities at their present level of performance. Yet it is equally important to continually raise the bar and encourage our kids, as they continue to make progress in their core deficit areas through traditional and compatible art therapy interventions. We do this so that they have the opportunity to continually make new choices as we raise the bar higher and higher. Is this easy for them or for us as parents, caregivers and professionals? Absolutely not.

Keri tells us about the frustrations of desperate, hair-pulling challenges parents, caregivers and professionals experience. Both as a mother and a professional in the field of autism, there were and still are times when she just wants to give up on raising the bar of expectation. It surely would be easier to just "do it for them?" wouldn't it? Or not? In Keri's words (2015):

> When my son was a child—and even now into adulthood, I am challenged and frustrated by attempting to teach the same thing over and over in an effort to help him improve his skills. Sometimes it just seems easier to do things for him rather than staying the course to support him to do things for himself, but in the end I know the quality of his life will suffer if I give in to this urge. Knowing I won't be there forever spurs me on to keep raising my bar for him despite my feelings of frustration or defeat.
>
> I see it as my job to help Taylor to be in the world as independently as possible before I pass on. If you are a parent, I have no doubt you have had a similar concept of the urgency to help your child to be "okay" after you are no longer here. We cannot help but feel this responsibility. It is our instinct to help our child to survive into adulthood.

When Taylor was eight years old, Keri wrote out a mission statement for his life:

> Taylor will live as independently as possible as an adult. He will receive the supports he needs to be successful and capable to the best of his best abilities. I will raise the bar of expectations for him to help him to achieve and accomplish these goals. Taylor will be loved and supported by those he loves and by those who love him.

When Taylor was one-and-a-half years old, Keri was told he might never walk or talk. At the time of writing Taylor is 27 years old and lives in his own apartment with limited weekly support. He still struggles with many things, but he has reached heights beyond all reason. Keri credits much of the support her son received as a child, which includes specific, constant and regular interventions in the arts.

THE URGENCY FOR QUALITY OF LIFE

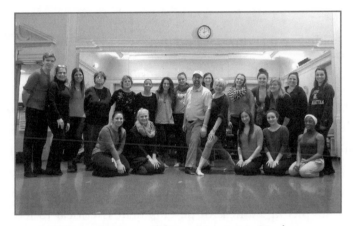

AMT certification workshop at Marymount Manhattan College, New York, NY, with Dr. Stephen M. Shore

Our urgent desire for our kids to have a better quality of life is what makes us raise the bar even when we are tired, frustrated, angry or lonely in our efforts. We know it can be excruciatingly painful for everyone involved to do over and over again the things that NT children often learn sooner, earlier and with less effort and less direct instruction. But what you see for your child's future must be your inspiration to do the hard work necessary, despite all the challenges. Refusing to give up on teaching fundamental skills is critical—knowing you are not alone is helpful. Seeing past the obstacles and frustrations of your efforts is equally important to gaining improvement and even mastery of specific skills. When you raise the bar and hold out expectations for your child, they will learn. Even when you do not experience your child as understanding or learning from your efforts, do not give up. There's a person in there listening and hearing you, despite appearances. Expect more and you will get more.

In too many instances where parents or professionals do not raise the bar, this has the appearance of defeat or of not understanding the importance of skill building; or perhaps it seems like the easiest path to just getting by. But this "easy" path becomes the one that children will pay dearly for as adults.

"It's just too hard for him," I hear parents say.

"There's just too many kids in my class to focus on one child," a teacher says.

"She will have a meltdown if I do that," says a caregiver.

And more commonly we hear, "You just don't understand."

Unfortunately, what we fail to pay for today, we will pay for exponentially in the child's future. Behavior and life skills are the first things that will determine a child's place in the world. What they learn as children—in behaviors, choice, life skills and eventually jobs—will determine their success as adults. Experience as a teacher has taught us that repetition in facilitating lessons in all areas of development is critical to learning new skills—even for those with limited or no language skills.

AMT is designed to cognitively redirect or re-map the brain through repetition of movement, patterns and sequences. For instance, in a 45-minute AMT class, the pattern and sequence we move to in Eric Bibb's song, "Don't Ever Let Nobody Drag Your Spirit Down" is the very same pattern and sequence performed in the second song we move to, "Fibre de Verre" by Paris Combo—both songs require cross-hemispheric body movement. Then at the end of the AMT class, we repeat the same pattern and sequence that we demonstrated in the first and second song to "Drop Me Off in New Orleans" by Kermit Ruffins.

This repetition of patterns and sequences establishes legitimate pathways or highways for the information to travel along, and the speed at which the brain can do that is amazingly fast. Go back to the analogy of moving to a new neighborhood; after a few trips to the grocery store, you do not have to turn on your GPS or get out your road map to make a quick run to the store for milk.

AUTISM MOVEMENT THERAPY: 45-MINUTE SESSION

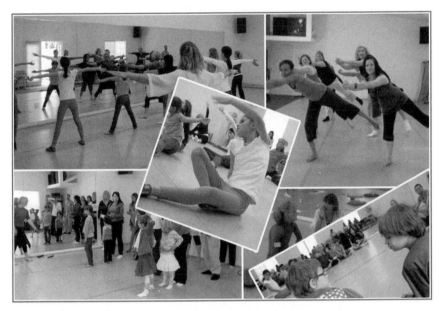

Montage of AMT classes

To get started, the direct prompt, "Everyone on your dot," is delivered by the instructor as the first AMT song, "Don't Ever Let Nobody Drag Your Spirit Down" is playing. The students should wear comfortable clothing that moves with the body. No shoes are required, but some kids who have sensory issues prefer to keep their socks on. Remember, socks can be slippery, so the bottoms of the socks can be either lightly sprinkled with water or ask the child to walk around outside in the socks to create some "dirt" traction.

Many teachers write to thank me for developing the AMT program. The teachers who do the AMT class in the classroom with their students leave the painter's tape on the floor so that the students are eager to begin each morning with the movement and music program. The teachers report to me increased social skills along with academic progress after incorporating AMT into the morning school schedule. Additionally, AMT leads to greater on-task activity, increased social skills awareness and ultimately behavioral challenge reduction allowing children the opportunity to be fully prepared to learn. The typical 45-minute class can be shortened, for example by only doing the first "Don't Ever Let Nobody Drag Your Spirit Down" and second "Fibre de Verre" songs and then finishing with the circle (outlined later in this chapter in more depth).

The goal of AMT is for the students' brains to respond to the re-mapping, with the ultimate goal of them being able to execute combinations independently, without the adult model, as the "how" transmitters are being reprogrammed.

Cognitive redirection or re-mapping requires dedication and perseverance, along with repetition and predictability, which are all keys to successful cross-hemispheric sensory integration. We want our kids to perform well and work on-task; mastering these basic skills can have an enormous impact in all other areas of learning. We also want them to be the best they can be. Autism Movement Therapy stimulates the brain and wakes up areas that have been dormant. But, like life, it's a process and no two kids respond in exactly the same manner. The program can be used with children as young as age three, yet has also been shown to be effective when started with teenagers and even adults. As we all say in our clinic "Don't get discouraged, get active! Retrain the brain!"

LET'S BREAK IT DOWN

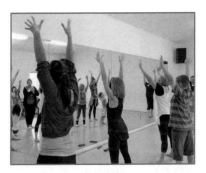

AUTISM MOVEMENT THERAPY (AMT): AMT is an empowering sensory integration strategy that combines music and movement to strengthen the left and right hemispheres of the brain. It combines patterning, visual movement calculation, audible receptive processing, rhythm, sequencing into a whole-brain cognitive thinking approach that can significantly improve behavioral, emotional, academic, social, speech and language skills

AMT class

You will need a CD player for the music or a sound system with a remote control to stop and start the music and to repeat the song when needed.

The six songs to use for the 45-minute AMT class are listed below, along with the movement that correlates to each one. Make sure to have the painter's tape on the floor to mark where the students should be standing as you begin the first two warm-up songs for the class.[1]

SONG 1: WARM-UP (7 MINS)

("DON'T EVER LET NOBODY DRAG YOUR SPIRIT DOWN" BY ERIC BIBB, MALI TO MEMPHIS, PUTUMAYO WORLD MUSIC)

If possible don't stop when the first song ends; go straight into the second song.

The foundation of AMT is the repetition of patterns and sequences, with the idea that the brain will remember the pattern and sequences of movement after it has been performed over the course of the class so that by the time we get to Song 6, we do the same pattern and sequence of movement as in Song 1 and 2. In Song 6, the tempo changes but the movement stays the same, the brain does not have to "think" where the body should be in space and what direction the body should move. The "cognitive mapping" of the pattern and sequence through repetition will allow the student to move through space

---

1   Thank you to Christina Jeremiah, Director Pipi Center Kuala Lumpers, Malaysia, for the "skills being taught" sections in this chapter.

with confidence and ease. (Attend an AMT Certification Workshop to learn AMT pattern and sequences designed for songs 1,2 and 6.)

SONG 2: HAND CROSSING (3.5 MINS)

("FIBRE DE VERRE" BY PARIS COMBO, FRENCH CAFÉ, PUTUMAYO WORLD MUSIC)

Lead students into the counting–hand crossing sequence. Clap hands on the thighs for two counts (1,2), then clap hands in front of the chest for two counts (3,4), push the hands out forward in front of the body for two counts (5,6), clap the hands on top of the head for two counts (7,8). Clap the hands in front of the body (midline) then extend the right hand out to the left, and the left hand out to the right for eight counts (repeat 4 times). Bring the arms up over the head, then down by the sides for eight counts. Then move into the same pattern and sequence from Song 1.

After this song, pause the music before the next portion.

SKILLS BEING TAUGHT (SONG 1 AND SONG 2)

1. Listening to cues.

2. Identifying:

   a. Left and right side

   b. Back and front

   c. Up and down.

3. Counting numbers 1–8 (recall).

4. Imitation skills.

5. Patterning-circle (basketball).

6. Sequencing receptive language.

7. Repetition.

8. Cross-movement (stimulates right and left brain—interhemispheric integration).

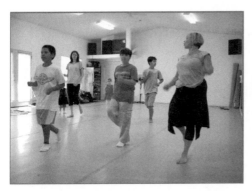 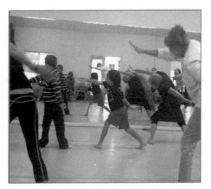

AMT warm up

CIRCLE TIME (20 MINS)

Ask the students to sit down on the floor in a circle, legs criss-cross applesauce (as in the picture below). The teacher leads the six Circle Floor Exercises (these are without music).

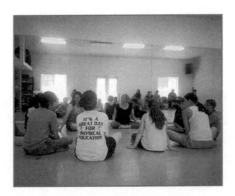

AMT Circle Time

1. FOUR MOVEMENTS AND FOUR SOUNDS (4 MINS)

The students sit on the floor in a circle. Each student leads (demonstrates) four movements with four sounds—the group reproduces the student's four movements and four sounds going around the circle. The student who has just led then touches the student to their left on the knee to let them know that they are the next leader who will demonstrate four movements and four sounds for the group. (Variation: the student who leads makes eye contact with another student to let that student know that they are now the leader.)

SKILLS BEING TAUGHT (FOUR MOVEMENTS AND FOUR SOUNDS)

1. Socialization with rules within a group.

2. Following a leader.

3. Listening to cues.

4. Turn taking.

5. Creative thinking—making movements and sounds (pairs gross motor with audio, visual processing and expressive language).

2. CLAPPING GAME (2 MINS)

This is the same as Four Movements and Four Sounds but movements and sounds are replaced with clapping a rhythm and the students repeat the rhythm. Go around the circle, using only a full physical prompt—no direct verbal instructions—pointing to each student with your palm sideways, your little finger pointing down and your arm outstretched (like a street-crossing guard). Each student in the circle has the opportunity to perform a clapping sequence that the other students will imitate.

3. THE NAME GAME (3 MINS)

Going around in the circle—one by one—each student stands up and divides their name into syllables, then executes one movement for each syllable in their name. The group in unison stands up and repeats that student's name, imitating the sequence of movements. Repeat this around the circle until each person has demonstrated their name and the group has imitated the movement, saying the name of the student as they perform the movement.

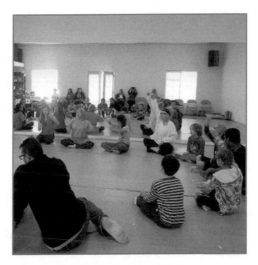

Keri leading Circle Time

SKILLS BEING TAUGHT (CLAPPING GAME AND THE NAME GAME)

1. Listening to cues.

2. Creative thinking—making sounds and movements for a name.

3. Eye contact.

4. Turn taking.

4. STORY DANCING (5–7 MINS)

The teacher begins on their right and proceeds around the circle so that each student has the opportunity to contribute one line to a sentence. For example, the teacher begins with a starter sentence, "I have a dog." The next student to the right repeats that sentence, and then adds a line to it. For example, "I have a dog and his name is Ben." The next student says, "I have a dog and his name is Ben and we like to play outside." Next student, "I have a dog and his name is Ben and we like to play outside and Ben chases the ball." Next student, "I have a dog and his name is Ben and we like to play outside and Ben chases the ball and Ben has four legs." Next student, "I have a dog and his name is Ben and we like to play outside and Ben chases the ball and Ben has four legs and he is black." (The key is for each student in turn to make eye contact with the student whose line they are repeating and adding on to.)

When there are five sentence ideas, and each student has participated with an additional line, the group stands up and begins to walk in a circle to the right, repeating all the sentences in unison as they move: "I have a dog, his name is Ben, we like to play outside, Ben chases the ball, Ben has four legs and he is black."

Stop the group, then reverse the direction to the left and repeat the entire sequence. Repeat until the group has walked in a circle two times to the right and two times to the left. Next, the group spreads out in the room—every student standing on a dot. The students begin to repeat all the sentences while adding movement. Make sure to use the entire dance floor and also make sure that the students have a beginning and an end—so, in other words, the sequence is discrete. This is Story Dancing.

5. ALPHABET CROSS-HEMISPHERIC CLAPPING (2 MINS)

Partners sit criss-cross applesauce facing one another. They clap in the middle of their body; then they reach across the midline of their body with their right hand to pat their partner's left hand and one of the partners says the letter A. They go back to center clap, then reach across the midline and pat their left hand against their partner's right hand and the "calling" partner says the letter B. They continue until all the letters of the alphabet have been said by one student; then the second student repeats the alphabet in the same manner.

SKILLS BEING TAUGHT (STORY DANCING AND ALPHABET CROSS-HEMISPHERE CLAPPING)

1. Eye contact.

2. Cross-clapping with partners (stimulates right and left brain).

3. Vocabulary is developed and improved.

4. Memory is improved.

5. Socialization with a partner.

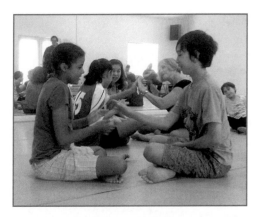

Alphabet cross-clapping

6. ANIMALS CROSS-HEMISPHERIC CLAPPING (2 MINS)

Partners sit criss-cross applesauce facing one another. Repeat the same sequence as in the Alphabet Cross-Hemispheric Clapping, but instead of saying the alphabet, the students name animals. This exercise switches from one student's turn to the other student's, so it is a "my turn, your turn" activity.

SONG 3: MOUSE (4 MINS)

("THE ADD-ON MACHINE" BY ERIC CHAPPELLE, MUSIC FOR CREATIVE DANCE, VOLUME 1)

The students line up in two parallel lines on the left side of the room. Designate two leaders. (Remember to put down tape as shown in the classroom diagram on page 46, and use painter's tape as visual markers for each student to stand on in a line behind the two designated line leaders.)

The teacher, to the beat of the music, says, "mouse cleaning hair" (while touching hair), "mouse cleaning ears," "mouse cleaning eyes," "mouse cleaning nose," "mouse cleaning cheeks" and so on until all the body parts on the next page have been identified:

- hair
- ears
- eyes
- nose

- cheeks
- mouth
- neck
- left shoulder

- right shoulder
- left elbow
- right elbow
- left knee

- right knee
- left foot
- right foot

SKILLS BEING TAUGHT (SONG 3)

1. Listening to cues.

2. Identifying body parts.

3. Counting and recall.

4. Following rhythm and patterns.

Next, motion for the students to wait and watch while you: demonstrate walking for four counts 1–2–3–4; do a half turn, 1, and freeze for three counts 2–3–4; continue across the floor until you have reached the other set of painter's tape markers.[2]

Now the students move across the floor in pairs repeating what you demonstrated: walk 1–2–3–4; half turn, 1 and freeze 2–3–4; walk 1–2–3–4; half turn, 1, and freeze 2–3–4.

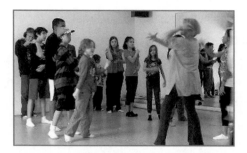

Mouse

---

2 Cross the floor once in each direction for the Mouse, the Elephant and the Slides. You may have to repeat the song (make sure you have a remote in your hand) if you have more than eight students in the class.

SONG 4: ELEPHANT

("ECHO LADY WHO" BY ERIC CHAPPELLE, MUSIC FOR CREATIVE DANCE, VOLUME 1)

The first pair of students begins from the first row marked with + from the left side of the room (see the AMT floor on page 46). Imitating an elephant walking, the arms being the trunk, they hop on their right leg towards the right with arms outstretched to the right and the left leg extended behind. Then they hop on the left leg towards the left with the right leg extended behind and the arms outstretched to the left (see the photo below). After each student has a turn going across the floor and has lined up on their dot in the row behind their leader then repeat the movement across the floor in the opposite direction.

SKILLS BEING TAUGHT (SONG 4)

1. Listening to cues.

2. Stimulating right and left brain.

3. Counting and recall.

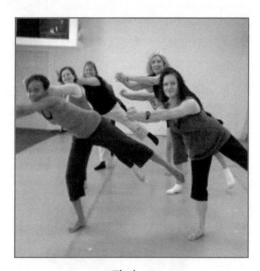

Elephant

SONG 5: SLIDES (6 MINS)

("CHIRPA, CHIRPA" BY ERIC CHAPPELLE, MUSIC FOR CREATIVE DANCE, VOLUME 1)

Two students at a time cross the floor with straight slides in each direction; they then add a half turn.

Variations include: students hold hands and cross the floor as partners; students hold hands and cross the floor circling; students skip across the floor; students cross the floor leading with their right leg and arms in second position, then the left leg leading with arms in second position.

SKILLS BEING TAUGHT (SONG 5)

1. Listening to cues.

2. Patterning.

3. Depending on a partner.

4. Eye contact.

5. Being single, then with partners.

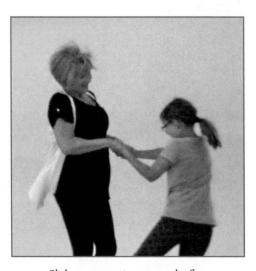

Slides—partnering across the floor

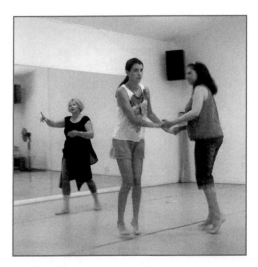

Partners slides across the floor

SONG 6: FREEZE DANCE (4.5 MINS)

("DROP ME OFF IN NEW ORLEANS" BY KERMIT RUFFINS, NEW ORLEANS, PUTUMAYO WORLD MUSIC)

The students move "free style" around the dance room to this Zydeco music. When the music stops, the students freeze. Choose a student and ask, "High, medium or low level?"

The student picks a level—for example, medium level. Now ask the student to choose between two imagination stances and pick one: "Softball player or horseback rider?" If the student chooses the softball player, everyone takes the medium-level softball player position and freezes. Make sure to call on all the students if you have a small group of 8–10 students.

Move to the center of the dance room and begin repeating the sequence from the Song 1, "Don't Ever Let Nobody Drag Your Spirit Down" in the warm-up (the sequence that was also repeated in the second song, "Fibre de Verre"). Let the students take a natural cue from you so that as you begin the warm-up the students should slowly move onto the dots that they were standing on at the beginning of the class.

Invite each student to lead for 8–16 counts in front of the class. "Jane, show us what to do." "Thank you. Ben, show us what to do." "Thank you. Sarah, show us what to do." And so on… Dance out the Zydeco music to the end.

SKILLS BEING TAUGHT (FREEZE DANCE)

1. Listening for natural cues—expressive movement.

2. Stimulating imagination.

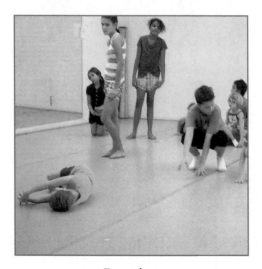

Freeze dance

IMAGINATION GAME (4 MINS)

The students lie in a circle on the floor after the Freeze Dance. Determine a location: beach, mountains, desert, etc. "Let's close our eyes and imagine we are at the beach... I see a pelican. What do you see, Andrew?" Ask each student what they see on the beach, and so on around the room until each student has been called on. If the student does not answer when you call on them, give them two choices to trigger an answer, for example, "Do you see a dolphin or a seagull?" The key here is to have the students bring a "visual picture image" to mind of what is being said. When each student has contributed, ask the students to roll over to their right sides and slowly come to a sitting position. Then proceed around the room asking each student what they saw on the beach during the exercise.

STEP BY STEP SUMMARY

- No music.

- Lead students to lie down on their backs on the floor.

- Ask students to close their eyes and breathe in and out slowly.

- Have one student choose a location where they want to be, for example, the beach or a mountain.

- Ask each student as they lie on the floor with their eyes closed, what they see (visualize) on the beach, for example, an umbrella, pelicans, ocean, dolphin.

- After each student has verbally revealed what they see (remember there is no right or wrong answer) ask them to slowly push up, placing their hands to the right side of their body and come to a sitting position.

- Go around the room and ask the students one by one to say again (recall) what they saw (imagined) in their mind.

SKILLS BEING TAUGHT (IMAGINATION GAME)

1. Using higher level cognitive thinking.

2. Recall.

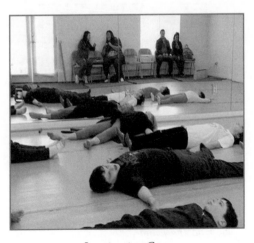

Imagination Game

SHOSHANA'S INCREDIBLE AMT JOURNEY FROM NO LANGUAGE TO SPEAKING

We asked Shoshana's mother to write for us what she thought we had accomplished as a team over the course of the past seven years in the AMT class. Below is what Andrea wrote verbatim.

> After taking our daughter to AMT for the past seven years the changes and/or improvements we have noticed are:
>
> 1. She is more complaint and willing to follow directions.
>
> 2. When we began, she was non-verbal; she now possesses functional speech and we are working on conversational speech.
>
> 3. Her focus and eye contact has improved and is still continuing to improve.
>
> 4. She now has an understanding of questions and short-term recall.
>
> 5. She is able to watch and process and imitate movements.
>
> 6. The other peers in the class she considers friends and enjoys seeing them every week.
>
> 7. Her father and I feel that AMT has helped Shoshana tremendously in also teaching us how to work with our daughter.

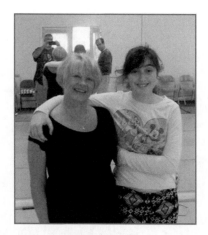

Shoshana and Joanne, 2015, in an AMT class

While there has been an enormous amount of measurable progress, we as a team will continue to raise the bar and ask Shoshana to rise to it. She is a young teen now, and as I look back over the past years of working with Shoshana, I see that: (1) she has friends; and (2) she is beginning to develop empathy and understanding for others on a level that far surpasses where she was seven years ago. When Shoshana was asked what she enjoyed best about the AMT class she told her mother Andrea: (1) Music (2) Exercise and (3) Ms. Lara. I couldn't have been more thrilled—first because she was able to organize; second, because she was able to list; and third, because I was included in the list!

In autism we have a term that is known as "Mindblindness" or "Theory of Mind" (TOM), the inability to understand what others may be thinking or feeling. Mindblindness, a term developed by Simon Baron-Cohen suggests, "Imagine what your world would be like if you were aware of physical things but were blind to the existence of mental things. Blind to things like thoughts, beliefs, knowledge, desires and intentions, which for most of us self-evidently underlie behavior (Baron-Cohen 1999, p.1).

Certainly, while some of Shoshana's progress can be attributed to natural maturation milestones, which, though late in developing, she has managed to meet, it is clear that Shoshana's brain has begun to process the variables in her environment at a higher level of cognitive thinking, this in turn allows her to analyse information which leads to higher level thinking skills. With this new level of thought, comes deduction and induction reasoning, through new cognitive pathways in the brain, for a whole thinking approach—i.e. Waking up the Brain!

CHAPTER 3

Music and Movement in Every Language

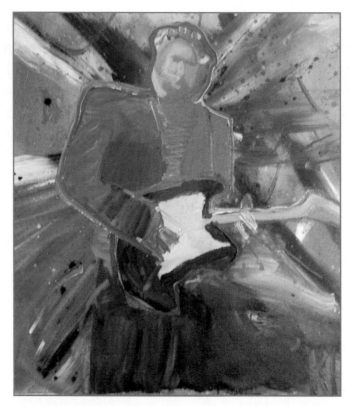

Art by Kevin Hosseini—Eric Clapton—the art of autism

"Musical training is a more potent instrument than any other, because rhythm and harmony find their way into the inward places of soul, on which they mightily fasten, imparting grace, and making the soul of him who is rightly educated graceful."

PLATO, THE REPUBLIC III CIRCA 387 B.C.

About a decade ago, when I was forming Autism Movement Therapy®, I came to a fork in the road. I could go two ways: One road was to speak and talk about environmental toxins that could possibly have a correlation to autism and the cause—I wrote my Master's thesis on "Environmental Toxins as an Etiological Factor in Autism"; or I could deliver hope and joy through movement and music to our families by providing a service that I knew to be successful because I had used a combination of the two in my Los Angeles Unified School District moderate/severe autism classrooms for years with amazing results. I made the latter career choice and I have not for one day been sorry.

I love my work, love bringing joy and happiness to others, especially when it is something that I feel so extremely passionate about in my own life! Everyone loves to DANCE! I have witnessed students who came to my class not talking, rolling on the floor and stimming on the classroom fluorescent ceiling lights, including one who left asking, "Will you be going to middle school with us Ms. Lara?" When I answered no, but that he could come anytime he liked and visit or call or email me, he replied, "We are going to miss you, Ms. Lara."

I watched this young man transition to working on computers and assisting in general education classrooms—all because of access to a strong music and movement program. We must raise the bar on our education system in this country and around the world. We must expect more, not less, from our kids, because they have autism and because the world outside both the classroom and the home will expect more from them, not less. We have to help our kids meet real-world challenges head-on so that they can become members of their communities, fall in love and have jobs! We should expect nothing less and it is our responsibility to make certain that we provide the educational environments that will prepare our students for just that. If it requires a kindergarten through secondary school social skills textbook curriculum that is facilitated by teachers and aides in the classroom on a weekly basis, then that is what governments and educators we need to provide. We must begin to meet the challenges and deficits of autism head on; and while we fill the gap in the social skills and language areas through the expressive arts, social skills curriculum and the PBS method, all the while we must support the students' strengths so that the challenges and deficits will meet in the middle and benefit the students in their future life and the real world.

WHAT WE KNOW ABOUT MUSIC

Music has the ability to transport our minds and redirect our thoughts, so it is important to choose the music in your home, office, car and classroom with care. Music and dance have the following benefits:

- Music and dance calm us and helps to regulate our moods.

- Dance and music have an enormous effect on our thinking and how we process information.

- We use all of our senses when we dance: our body, our ears and our eyes.

- Most important of all: we use our *"whole brain"* when we dance.

- It allows for increased inclusion opportunities.

- Music and dance provide an excellent platform to teach social studies, that is, cultural diversity through music and dance.

- Movement and music is universal language.

- Dance and Music add an element of beauty to our life.

- We do not need to communicate verbally when we dance.

- Dancing to music engages both the left and right hemispheres of the brain.

Torres and Donnellan tell us:

All too often in the case of autism and other disorders of the nervous system, the affected individual is treated in third person and dehumanized. Here an active effort was made to open the conversation to those who experience what it is like to live day to day with this disorder and to the parents, caregivers and others who advocate for them. As researchers, our relationships with autistic individuals and their families need to change. Likewise, the science behind autism research also needs a radical transformation if we aim at succeeding in this effort. The field needs to take a cross-disciplinary approach to this very complex phenomenon.

There are ingenious solutions in each autistic nervous system that biology has already found to cope with the disorder. We need to tune in and learn to understand those biological solutions. We need to support the person with many accommodations. We need to work together with the overarching goals of inclusion and presumed competences to truly lighten the burdens as well as acknowledge the strengths and possibilities that autism creates for the individual (Torres and Donnellan 2015).

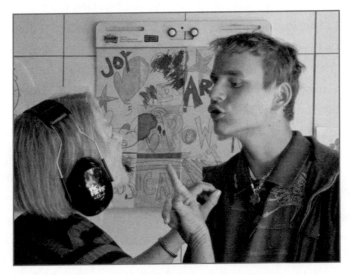

Joanne and Neal

In the photograph above, Neal and I are speaking after an AMT session during an Expressive Arts Camp made possible by an Autism Speaks Grant. Typically, Neal would insist on the headphones being on his head but he agreed to allow me to wear them so long as he could see them.

Temple Grandin tells us in the documentary *Generation A: Portraits of Autism and the Arts* that music is processed in a different "circuit" of the brain, which is why some kids can sing before they can talk. Enough cannot be said about the importance of allowing our children access to a strong school-based music program along with a wide choice of musical instruments. As parents and advocates, you may want to push a little harder at the next team meeting, and do not take "No" for an answer when you ask if your child can be fully included with the general education students in the music class at school. Often times we find that the public schools are reluctant to accept our students with severe autism—the very kiddos who will benefit the greatest from a strong structured music program, if we are to embrace what Dr. Grandin says.

Dr. Stephen M. Shore, advocate, Associate Professor at Adelphi University and self-professed individual with Asperger's explains, "Whatever seems to scramble the speech centers of the brain tends to leave the music areas intact" (Shore 2002). Stephen says that when he gives private music lessons to individuals across the autism spectrum, he finds that the music promotes communication in one of three ways: First, for those individuals who are preverbal or have not developed a reliable means of communication, music can be *the* means of communicative interaction. Second, for others, music helps promote existing verbal communication. "I've had students who are functionally nonverbal yet they can sing with perfect diction and pitch," Stephen says, supporting Temple Grandin's statement. Third, for another subset of the population, music may serve as a sort of carrier signal that helps organize communication. Interestingly, as with all of humanity, some of Dr. Shore's students have the skill and ability to become professional musicians. Others have to work harder at music but still enjoy the process. Finally, much as he doesn't like to admit, there are some individuals whom he says, "I have yet to figure out how to reach."

In addition to the therapeutic benefits of music Dr. Shore chooses to give music lessons to individuals with autism because it provides a real life skill in which to develop interactions with others as a soloist or member of a musical ensemble. Since he has not figured out how to teach NT children, he just sticks with those on the autism spectrum, who, he explains, make much more sense to him.

One father at a recent "Sweet 16" birthday party for a young teenager on the spectrum gloats, "My son loves to listen to music and dance around," a statement heard more often than not, usually from parents of newly diagnosed children with autism spectrum disorder (ASD). We want to look closely and truly honor what the child is really communicating to us: he not only finds comfort in music and moving his body but he also is likely to be using the movement and music to regulate himself in his environment as well.

Another father at the same party beams as he tell us that his 17-year-old son with very limited communication skills always loved music as a child and danced around the living room with earphones and an iPod. Jokingly, the father adds, "I probably owe a great deal of gratitude to Steve Jobs, iPods, iPads and Apple in general." When pressed, "Does your son play a musical instrument?" the father smiles proudly and answers, "Yes, the clarinet."

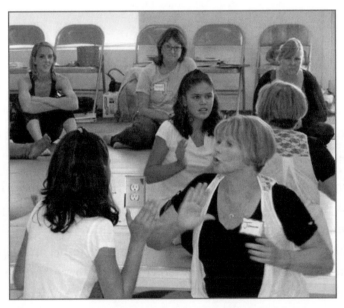

Joanne and a student in an AMT Certification Workshop

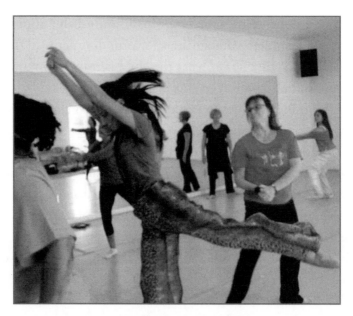

AMT certification workshop

PIANIST TIMOTHY DRURY ON MUSIC IS MATH

Timothy Drury played with Don Henley as a member of the band for 11 years, was a regular guest pianist for the Eagles and was a member of the band Whitesnake as the keyboard player. When he was asked his thoughts on the statement, 'music is math' he replied:

> When I was first starting to play and learn how to read music, I suppose it was much more about numbers and note values, but as I grew and became more articulate with my fingers, it was the SHAPES that my hands and fingers were making as they were playing a particular progression or chord that I was remembering, not the numeric values, and that is what has stuck with me ever since. I see various types of triangles, arrows, vectors, parallelograms. They appear on the keyboard and make a strong visual impression in my mind. My brain stores these shapes, I suppose, to be accessed at will as I'm playing. Each shape represents a particular sound, mood, feeling. THAT particular process, which occurs each moment I'm playing, is a complete mystery to me, but I'm quite happy to have this mnemonic system in place, and it

seems to have served me well over the years. Oh, and by the way, I still have never, EVER, used Algebra for any reason, at any time, in my adult life. (2014)

Fascinating!

What does all this mean? Temple Grandine, Dr. Shore and Timothy Drury are all speaking about the same idea that the brain processes information in our environment in sometimes varied and different ways. While the job of each of the four lobes remains consistent, the information processing itself is where we will focus, as it is the very essence of what the term "gifted" means. We use this word when referring to individuals who excel in one particular area of expertise. Individuals with autism have what we call "splintered skill sets," and they are many times gifted in these skill set areas. Social and behavior may remain as challenge domains but activities in which they may excel include computer graphics, animation, playing a musical instrument such as the cello or guitar, singing…the list goes on and on.

The process of how the brain "listens to music" has been studied in depth over the past decade. The well-known physician, scientist and author Oliver Sacks explains in his book *Musicophilia: Tales of Music and the Brain* (2007) that the magic of music illuminates the strange workings and misfirings, of the human mind. Lauren Stewart tells us that the brain changes after learning to read and play music:

> The study of the brain bases for normal musical listening has advanced greatly in the last 30 years. The evidence from basic and clinical neuroscience suggests that listening to music involves many cognitive components. Using patient cases reported in the literature, we develop an approach for understanding disordered musical listening that is based on the systematic assessment of the perceptual and cognitive analysis of music and its emotional effect. This approach can be applied both to acquired and congenital deficits of musical listening, and to aberrant listening in patients with musical hallucinations. Both the bases for normal musical listening and the clinical assessment of disorders now have a solid grounding in systems neuroscience. (Stewart *et al.* 2006, p.11)

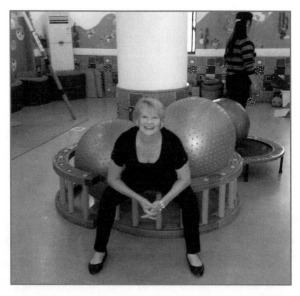

Joanne Lara in autism preschool sensory room, Nanjing, China

CHINA AND MUSIC

In the fall of 2014, Keri and I were given the opportunity to present an impromptu AMT session to a group of 25 preschool children at a small autism center in Nanjing, China. We had both been invited to speak at the International Autism Conference held in the eastern city of Nanjing. When we arrived at the school, we entered with uncertainty—unsure of what to expect from our visit. We had not been given instructions and/or requests for a particular orientation or demonstration in advance; we had been merely asked to teach a "a music and movement" class for 20 or so preschoolers, so we were on our own to take control of the situation and forge ahead with our lesson plan.

The room was buzzing with chaotic anticipation. The children, who were seated in neat rows on tiny plastic chairs, were visibly distressed, crying and whining, their morning routine having been disrupted by both our attendance, and by their parents' presence in the room. Typically, the parents were not at the school during the school sessions, but today the eager moms and dads had been invited to see the "ladies from Los Angeles who dance with children." We purposefully noted the chaos and distress in the kids, and pointed out how the room was arranged (theater style) to make a particular point.

As is often the case in autism, we find our best-laid plans become disrupted and things do not go according to schedules or expectations. When this happens, the best idea is to improvise in the moment and get things moving. No doubt, you have experienced behaviors or circumstances that disrupt your daily lives on a regular basis. This can be radically magnified for an autistic child. We find that when we breathe into the unexpected instead of letting the "problem" overcome us, we can take more positive actions to transform our challenges. We like to say there are no problems—we simply have situations in need of a solution. This was our mission on that particular morning.

Seeing the disorder in the room, we looked at one another and knew instantly what we needed to do. "We've got to take charge of this situation. I'll move the chairs, you help move the kiddos into place." We were soldiers on a mission, working in tandem to organize the chaos. With dozens of children and adults in the room, calm intention and actions were our primary goal. Hurriedly, we rearranged the room, moving the chairs to the outer parameters of the space to make a larger space in the center of the room to dance with three- and four-year-olds.

In order to facilitate AMT, it is necessary to have an area in which to move from one side of the room to the other side in a straight line in pairs. Whether facilitating AMT with one child or a group of participants, the value of the AMT structured processes of connection, imitation, leadership, trust and expression are at the core of the methodology.

As we moved the chairs away from the center of the room, we motioned to the parents to take a seat in the little chairs and put their children (criss-cross applesauce) on the floor in front of them. The parents seemed more confused by this than the children—*shouldn't children sit properly in chairs?* When the kids finally sat down, they almost immediately began to calm down, and we watched as the chaos turned to relative calm.

Imitating the beat of our hearts

We began our session without a conventional greeting or introduction. Instead, we jumped right into our session with two beats on our improvised drums—large Lego® blocks turned upside down that we found in the corner of the room. Simultaneously, we chanted (sang) "*Nĭ hăo Nĭ hăo*," the standard greeting for "hello" in Chinese, but which literally means "You good." We gave no verbal prompt for the children to repeat our initial two beats (greeting) but instead pointed to the children themselves as a visual prompt and then pointed to their Lego blocks to indicate that it was now their turn.

We had asked Lavender, our Chinese translator, to hold off relaying any of our instructions in Chinese. We wanted the children, parents and staff to see, hear, and intuit our request to imitate our actions through "non-verbal" communication—save the greeting, "*Nĭ hăo*."

Imitation, where the observer repeats another's actions is a primary principal of ABA. The highest form of social learning, and how humans and animals teach all new skills to their young, imitation involves a child's ability to copy people's actions—in this case, drumming on Lego blocks while singing the greeting. Researchers who have studied the abilities of children with autism to mimic or imitate have found that the early ability to imitate gestures and body movements predicts language outcomes (Toth *et al.* 2006).

Imitation is also related to joint attention (the ability to share a focus with another person on an activity or object) and directly affects social, life and play skills; so we know that direct lessons in teaching imitation skills is essential to developing a variety of critical skills that the individual will use throughout their life. The AMT experience is designed with this objective in mind.

Because the very nature of AMT is fun, relaxed and enjoyable, we see that kids readily loosen up and become more receptive and capable of building imitative skills. That morning session was no exception. As expected, our visual and sing-song prompts immediately showed results. One little boy, who innately understood what to do, repeated the beats and words with perfect precision. His father, who was sitting behind him, beamed with pride while joining in with the fun. So, too, did a few of the other parents who were sitting behind their children and their makeshift Lego block drums.

Carrying on, with three syllable beats, we sang (now in English,) "Good mor-ning," while simultaneously demonstrating three beats on our drums which matched the syllables of the greeting. Again, with no verbal prompting, we pointed to the children and their drums. This time, a few more children understood and intuited our greeting and drum beats and repeated our demonstration. Prompted by the visuals and sounds, they were able to tune into the tempo, rhythm and intonation of the musical drumbeats and sing-song words we modeled.

In addition to imitation, in a regular AMT session, we also include a broad range of activities and opportunities for the children to lead, prompt and design their own actions for others, as we learned in Chapter 2. During Circle Time "Four Movement and Four Sounds," "Clapping Game" and "Story Dancing" all use this primary technique. Unfortunately, in this short session, due to time restraints we were unable to build this activity into the class, but leadership and developing imagination are fundamental to developing higher-level thinking skills. ("Does your child have imagination skills?" is a question near the center of one of the initial assessment tools, the ADI™-R, used globally to determine eligibility of autism (Rutter *et al.* 2005, p.21).

BOX 3.1 GOOD VIBRATIONS

The bass of drum beats is felt in the body. Even when functional language is absent, or when a child appears not to understand or hear us, their body feels the vibration and rhythm of the beats. You will have experienced this before. For example, when the bass of music is heard through a wall, or when a car passes you with loud, rock or hip hop music blaring from its interior, you can feel the sound in your body. As you have likely noticed, the beat of the bass you feel gains your full attention. You are aware you can feel the beat. Our drum beats and greeting served the same purpose. It gained the attention of the children's body and mind. Music is strong, powerful "stuff," the universal source of communication for all mankind. Early primal communication with the cave man took place through drum-talking, where the drums signalled danger and occasions for celebration, death and birth.

Show me, don't tell me

As the children followed our lead, they also followed one another. Many of them looked about the room at what their peers were doing and followed suit. Smiles grew wider and attention increased. A couple of the kiddos, not yet able to follow the rhythm, were banging sporadically with hard, rapid beats on the Lego blocks. When this happens—as it will tend to do in AMT sessions when children become overwhelmed by the music, the beat, and the idea that they themselves are the source—a key factor in AMT is that we honor anything that the student imitates, even if it is not what has been demonstrated. We are teaching discreteness: that things in our life have a beginning, a middle and an end. Many of our children with severe autism are at the mercy of their brain, which is moving a thousand miles an hour; and if a child is sensory seeking, they are not aware that behaviors, ideas and thoughts have a beginning, a middle, and an end. This accounts for why so many of our kids with attention deficit hyperactivity disorder (ADHD) want to continually move their bodies in space, circling and spinning to self-regulate.

So, for example, if a child, during "Four Movement and Four Sounds" is shy and doesn't want to participate, we honor that child by doing whatever movement and/or sound the student did discretely. In other words, if the child looked down at their foot and grabbed their toes, then we look down at our feet and grab our toes, making certain to give the entire movement a beginning, a middle and an end and that we all physically replicate what the child has done. In this way we honor the child and they feel worthy. It is amazing to see the child's face when they realize that all the other students are doing what they did. Think about it, our kids with disabilities are so rarely held up as models. The times are few and far between when students with autism are asked to come up to the front of the class and show the other students how to do something. The bottom line is that they are often not comfortable in a leadership role. At the end of each AMT class we ask each student to come up to the front as "Drop Me Off in New Orleans" is playing and "show us how to do it." Each student has the opportunity to lead the class in their chosen movement; there is no wrong or right way, so whatever the student does, we follow (imitate) as a group.

In the case of this preschool class in China, while still sitting on the floor, facing the students with legs crossed, a simple verbal prompt was given: "We hit the drum like this…" Then we again modeled the desired beat and repeated the verbal greeting. One little girl, who had greater challenges in her ability to imitate and pay attention, was banging her Lego drum hard and loud. Another simple prompt was given: "Can I see your pretty eyes?" She stopped the banging and looked up, then down again, and proceeded to continue banging on the drum. Calmly, a second verbal prompt was given along with a full physical demonstration (actually modeling the drum beat), saying, "Like this…"

A very important value of AMT is that the children (or adults) motor their own actions. In other words, we do not drag children by the hand, tug on shirts and so on, to prompt imitation. We seek to make eye contact, model the desired actions and encourage independent self-determination skills (see Box 3.2). Although it is rare for us to use hand-over hand facilitation in AMT, in the case of this little girl, after three attempts to support her in imitating the beats with no success, hand-over-hand (actually placing your hands on the hands of the child and motoring the child through the skill) instruction was used. With that, she was able to model the correct beats—albeit for only a short period of time—before she began to bang on the Lego drum again. No worries, we were successful in our attempt for her to initiate the sought-after skill, even if only for a short period of time; now we could build on that independent response in the future and extend the time spent on that task. This is how we do it: We teach the skill without motoring the child through it and train the brain to "wake up!" in the process.

Unfortunately, we were unable in that session to work one-on-one with the girl and a few other children who would have benefited from more personal attention. But we ask you this: if she could imitate our actions just once, for a short period of time, imagine what her progress would be over a period of days, weeks or months. With continued, dedicated imitation instruction, might she improve these valuable skills? How would more time and practice increase her attention span? We continued with our lesson…

"One plus one is two!" (with five beats). Now most of the children and parents were joining in.

"Two plus two is four!" (five more beats on our Lego drum). We then added more complex drum beats.

"My name is Jo-anne, I like to dance!" (nine simultaneous beats).

"My name is Ker-i, I like mu-sic!" (nine beats).

The vibration in the room rose as the preschoolers and parents smiled and laughed more assuredly while echoing the rhythms, beats and sing-song words with impressive accuracy. As the expression of joy rose, it was evident that the parents and staff began to understand with their own eyes, ears and bodies, what no words were necessary to describe. Music and movement wakes up the brain!

BOX 3.2 STOP TUGGING, PULLING AND PHYSICALLY MOTORING YOUR CHILD!

There is a common universal theme with many parents of autistic children: an instinct (or desire) to "force" compliance or action by physical manipulation. In virtually every culture, we tend to take autistic children (and adults) by the hand, tug on shirts, and push or pull them into forced action. This inevitably creates the opposite effect. What we really want to see is independence and self-determination. If we want our children to learn to self-monitor and generalize the necessary skills, they must do it on their own after we have directly instructed them. For example, if a child falls to the floor and will not get up unless an adult or caregiver pulls them up, over time they become dependent upon someone picking them up. This serves to reinforce the behavior of falling to the floor most likely as an attention-seeking or escape avoidance behavior. We will discuss the four functions of behavior in Chapter 4.

Changing old ideas into new possibilities— I like the way you're thinking!

The concept of movement, music and the arts as tools to develop essential skills is an entirely new concept for many parents and professionals. It certainly was for those parents in China, whose cultural values and ideas of education are rooted in excellence in academics, performance and the "proper" conduct of children. The culture of autism in many countries around the world remains years behind more progressive nations, where floor time, self-determination, self-expression and meeting children "where they are" are valued. Yet even in the United States, Canada, Europe and other advanced countries, we still see a reluctance to embrace the arts. Though this is changing, the arts are still considered merely as enrichment or a "nice" thing to do. The arts are not yet considered essential or vital as powerful tools of opportunity. And yet, anecdotally, we see that when AMT (and other arts) are facilitated with a clear goal, objective and outcome in mind, powerful results are seen. And when we "see" these beneficial outcomes for ourselves we become believers.

It is hard to dismiss an intervention that supports a child's first words; one that allows the child to becomes less anxious; or one that enables a child to stand in front of the door eager to leave their house to go to a Saturday AMT class. That is the beauty of AMT, where benefits are often seen in the first session, as was the case in China.

For the second half hour of our class that day, we moved on to the dance portion of the class. Finally, we were ready to have Lavender interpret other important core messages of AMT's movement and music methods. The following instructions and values were repeated for the group in Chinese.

We went on to instruct, "Everybody on your dot!" This is where visual prompts become an important tool. As explained in Chapter 2, we always put blue or white painter's tape on the floor prior to the students' arrival to mark the spots where they should stand. The dot signifies where their physical bodies should be in the room as well as serving as a reminder to "wake up the brain." The students asking themselves, "Where is my place in this room?" is the key, not you showing them where they should be. We are careful to let the students locate and go to their own dot in the room—you want to avoid taking them by the hand and leading them to a dot on the floor unless it is their first time in the dance space. Remember, we always want to promote independence and self-determination skills that lead to higher-level thinking that can be generalized to other settings in the student's life (i.e. "Where is my place in this setting, this room, this environment and the world").

Within minutes, we had the children moving across the floor, mimicking animal movements (the Mouse and the Elephant), skipping, turning, partnering and holding hands (facing one another) to slide across the floor in pairs. For some, just moving their bodies from one side of the room to the other was the lesson. AMT finds children "where they are" and then raises the bar of expectation over time! This is an important key principal of AMT.

BOX 3.3 HE CAN'T TALK, BUT HE CAN SING!

"In autism, there are deficits on the left side of the brain whose job it is to interpret and administrate speech—whereas music and singing is interpreted on the right side of the brain (Grandin 2013, p.91). This may explain, as Temple Grandin tells us, why some children who do not have functional language can sing a song."

While music and speech seem very different, they have in common tempo, rhythm and intonation and require the use of the same phonotory and articulatory brain mechanisms (Sacks 2007). Is it the tempo, rhythm and intonation interpreted on the right side of the brain that helps to build a bridge to the left side of the brain through the corpus callosum, which then connects and supports the development of language?

Expectations accomplished

To close the session, we modeled putting the blocks away (clearing up) by stacking a few Lego blocks against the wall, and then pointed to the children to do the same, motioning from parents and assistants to pull back and let the child do it alone—independently. One by one, those itsy-bitsy kiddos picked up their Lego blocks, walked across the room, and stacked them neatly as the child before them had modeled. Lavender translated into Chinese that the skill of stacking blocks served to increase fine and gross motor skills, social and life skills, and self-determination.

The happy tears we saw in the eyes of the parents as they watched their children place their Lego blocks neatly on the stack told us that they understood our methods, and one more thing—that their children could interpret and imitate when constructive and meaningful lessons were taught. This would be confirmed by emails we received from several parents who wrote to share their experiences that day.

Presume competence

Lavender translated the following:

> Presume competence. Even if your child has no language, know they are hearing you. They are listening even when we think they do not hear us. This is evidenced by individuals who as adults found facilitated communication through technology (another art form we think); and now children who communicate using iPads tell us to the effect: "When you thought I wasn't listening, I heard every word you said."

One email in particular, received from the mother of David, is important and thought-provoking on many levels. *Note: Her first language is Chinese. We have not changed her grammar and share it as written.*

> Before my son David was recently diagnosed with autism, I sometimes disliked him for he changed from a very good boy (He was a very good boy before two, and then started to change gradually) into such a naughty one who gave me a lot of headaches. I sometimes lost my patience, so I yelled at him and even punished him. You can't tell him how regretful I am now. After the diagnosis, I came to know the reasons what made him change and his so-called bad behavior was not what he can control. But your speech enabled me to share his feelings and understand him better. After your speech, my eyes were filled with tears whenever I think of what sufferings he has gone through. Oh, my poor son…

When we presume competence and raise the bar of expectations, we see that even small children can learn important life skills. By modeling patience and commitment to the processes, new skills can and will be learned. For example, even a small child can learn to pick up and put away their own toys or clothes, and take their plate from the table to the sink. But we need to model the steps or use a task analysis chart placing photos of the child (or use PECS icons) doing the skill in the incremental order that the skill is learned, meaning discretely with a beginning and an end. As the skill is being taught, the adult can point to the photo of where the child is in the skill-task breakdown to help prompt the child as to what comes next. (Remember to use hand-over-hand only when absolutely necessary to accomplish the task.)

Teaching life skills to a small child with autism can surely be unnerving. The challenges of teaching these skills can make us want to pull our hair out at times. In our fast-paced lives, it's just easier to do it for them, right? Wrong! Make no mistake. What we do not invest in today, we and our children will pay for dearly later on in life. We must raise our expectations early on if we hope one day to see our children become more capable, independent adults. If we wait until later; until it is easier; until we have time; until, until, until…we are wasting precious time on dependency instead of self-determination, and we are not ultimately serving our child or their future.

ROCKING TO THE BEAT—INTERESTING FACTS ABOUT MUSIC

Did you know that monkeys can't tap their feet to songs, or recognize beats? It appears that humans are the only primates that move to the beat of music. In Landau's 2012 CNN documentary *Music: It's in your head, changing your brain,* Aniruddh Patel at the Neurosciences Institute in San Diego, California, speculates that this is because our brains are organized in a different way than our close species relatives. Grooving to a beat may be related to the fact that no other primates can mimic complex sounds (Landau 2012).

Curiously, some birds can mimic what they hear and move to beats. Patel's research with a cockatoo suggests the beat responses may have originated as a byproduct of vocal mimicry, but also play a role in social bonding (Patel in Landau 2012). Armies train by marching to a beat, for instance. Group dancing is a social activity. Studies also show that when people move together to a beat, they're more likely to cooperate with each other in non-musical tasks than if they're not in sync. Patel said, "Some people have theorized that that was the original function of this behavior in evolution: it was a way of bonding people emotionally together in groups, through shared movement and shared experience" (Patel in Landau 2012).

Another exciting arena of research—music with a beat seems to help people with motor disorders, such as Parkinson's disease, walk better than in the absence of music—patients actually synchronize their movements to a beat, Patel added "That's a very powerful circuit in the brain," he said in Landaus 2012 documentary, "It can actually help people that have these serious neurological diseases."

There's also some evidence to suggest that music can help Alzheimer's patients remember things better, and that learning new skills such as musical instruments might even stave off dementia.

There still needs to be more research in these areas to confirm, but Charles Limb, associate professor of otolaryngology and head and neck surgery at Johns Hopkins University, is hopeful about the prospect of musical engagement as a way to prevent, or at least delay, dementia. "That's a pretty amazing thing that, from sound, you can stimulate the entire brain," Limb said (Landau 2012). "If you think about dementia as the opposite trend, of the brain atrophying, I think there's a lot of basis to it" (Limb in Landau 2012).

MUSIC IS MATH—SUMMING IT UP!

> "Music is the pleasure the human mind experiences from counting without being aware that it is counting."
>
> GOTTFRIED LEIBNIZ CIRCA 1679

Music, with all of its emotional and creative passion, is based upon both simple and complex mathematical relationships. The similarities between music and math includes numbers, patterns, measurements, proportions, ratios and geometry. Musical notions including chords, scales, keys and octaves can all be understood using simple math. As numbers have rhythms and patterns, so too does music. We have heard it said that modern mathematics is "the basis of sound" and "sound itself" in its musical aspects.

The patterns that govern music and math can be looked at by thinking of a guitar. Each fret on a guitar—frets are numbered just like strings by the space in-between the metal pieces (or bridges)—raises the pitch of the string by one semi-tone. This rise is due to the mathematical relationship between the original length of the string, the amount by which it was shortened, and the resulting rise in pitch. This rise in pitch has a lot to do with ratios.

So why should we care if music is math? The answer is as complex as it is simple: predictability. In autism, one of the core assets and, conversely, one of the core deficits can be the need for predictability, routine, sameness. If a child can predict, they can relax. If they can relax, they can learn better. Music—and dance—as a "Golden Ratio" provides this predictability in their world.

For this reason, we might draw the conclusion that math and music, in their mutual predictabilities, are what draw many autistics to music, math, science and technology. Even those autistics with greater behavior challenges are drawn to music. Such was the case with Albert Einstein, who is believed to have an ASD. Einstein had significantly delayed speech as a child, and, at times, difficulties with language as an adult. He was challenged by social interactions, and had tactile/sensory issues. Yet, Einstein, who loved music deeply, was perhaps the most brilliant mathematician of all times. He is known to have said that his passion for music was extraordinarily helpful to him in his work (Mahadevan 2015).

In the NT population, we know for sure that music education has a clear and meaningful impact on mathematical development. We also know that music supports the development of critical skills such as listening, turn taking, patience, fine motor skills, problem solving, and so on. Studies are beginning to see a similar impact in individuals with autism. Dr. Stephen Shore reiterates, "Early exposure to keyboard music increases the neural connection in the corpus callosum. Since the corpus callosum is often smaller/thinner in those with autism, it's a 'no-brainer' (pun intended) to teach music to people on the autism spectrum" (2014).

PART II

BEHAVIOR–BEHAVIOR–BEHAVIOR AND THE VALUE OF TEACHING SOCIAL SKILLS

CHAPTER 4

Behavior–Behavior–Behavior

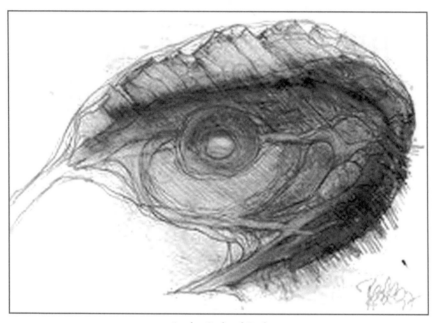

Art by Gerhard Beck

"It's nice to respect, be polite, do what you're asked to do and follow directions because you will have more friends and people will want to play with you."

SOPHIA ROSE BATHUM, 10 YEARS OLD

This chapter will take the reader through the process of understanding that behavior is meaningful for the individual, has a function and can be addressed through Positive Behavior Support (PBS).

People display behavior every second, hour and minute of the day by breathing, walking, running…dancing. The goal for unacceptable behavior that is socially inappropriate and not going to serve the individual well is to redirect the socially unacceptable behavior and teach replacement skills in place of the inappropriate behavior in order for the individual to be successful. PBS emphasizes respecting, valuing, dignifying, understanding and listening to individuals who may display "behavior problems."

The four different functions of behavior for all individuals will be explored in this chapter, as well as PBS strategies. In order to provide appropriate learning environments, including the dancefloor, classroom and community, which are supportive and creative for the individual, we want to positively reward them for behavior that we want to see again and again over time.

WHAT SHOULD A BEHAVIOR PLAN LOOK LIKE?
TOOLS FOR CHALLENGING BEHAVIORS

One of the primary core challenges of a diagnosis of autism manifests in the area of behavior. Early behavioral intervention strategies can dramatically increase the quality of life for individuals with ASD by enhancing the possibilities of increased educational, social, and independent or supported living skills.

Educators, therapists and researchers agree that consistent early intervention is the key to remediating problem behaviors in individuals with ASD. Behavior Analysis is the science of behavior and Applied Behavior Analysis (ABA) refers to a systematic and scientific approach to the assessment and evaluation of behavior, and the applications of interventions such as PBS to alter these behaviors. ABA is a *methodology* used to teach new skills and PBS is a *strategy* used to modify behaviors that are unwanted by reinforcing appropriate behavior. Punishments such as "benching" and "time out" are not used as strategies in PBS but are found in the ABA method.

What studies indicate, is that when PBS strategies are implemented early on, the individual benefits greatly by an overall "increased quality of life." Behavior issues make it difficult to make and maintain friends; after leaving the school setting, individuals with ASD often find themselves in the spare back room of their family home, alone, without friends, watching DVDs or sitting at the computer day in and day out. Mainstreaming and full inclusion do not guarantee friends, as many children, even after being mainstreamed or fully included, often lack the social skills to sustain the friendships that would normally travel with them throughout their academic lives and on into their post-academic living quarters and workplaces. Negative or disruptive behaviors in the home and school setting in the early years distance our children from their peers, impeding and limiting their ability to ultimately make and keep friends.

WHAT IS POSITIVE BEHAVIOR SUPPORT?

The Individual with Disabilities Education Act (IDEA) is a US federal law that requires schools to serve the educational needs of eligible students with disabilities. According to IDEA '97, PBS is the recommended form of intervention for dealing with challenging behavior in children with disabilities (Cohn 2011). Andrea M. Cohn of the National Association of School Psychologists defines PBS as follows:

> Positive Behavioral Support (PBS) is an empirically validated, function-based approach to eliminate challenging behaviors and replace them with prosocial skills. Use of PBS decreases the need for more intrusive or aversive interventions (i.e., punishment or suspension) and can lead to both systemic as well as individualized change. (Cohn 2001)

First and foremost, in order to address a behavioral plan for a student we must know what the function of the behavior is for that specific individual in the specific environmental setting that the behavior occurs.

DETERMINING THE FUNCTION OF THE BEHAVIOR

Despite IDEA calling for PBS to be used with ASD students, in many cases, it is not. Often times, staff have not been properly trained in the implementation of the strategies, and usually even those who have been trained find it difficult to put the concepts into practice when they are confronted with challenging behavior in a real-life, everyday situation. PBS is the only IDEA behavioral intervention strategy specifically "required" for behavioral management. It has long been a component of IDEA because it is a simple, direct, ideological method that works. A behavioral intervention plan (BIP) is designed for a specific child to try to help them learn to change their behavior. Once the function of a student's behavior has been determined, the Individual Education Program (IEP) team should develop the behavior intervention plan.

There are a number of ways to determine the function of a behavior. The tool most often used is the Motivational Assessment Scale (MAS), developed by Dr. V. Mark Durand and Dr. Daniel B. Crimmins (Durand and Crimmins 1992). Functional communication training is an empirically validated approach to PBS for challenging behavior (Durand and Merges 2001).

A simple and easy-to-use tool, the MAS is a quick way of understanding the purpose underlying the problem behavior. The purpose or function for the behavior is broken down into four main categories:

1. attention-seeking behavior

2. avoidance or escape behavior

3. tangible/to get something behavior

4. sensory/it feels good behavior.

Once we have determined the function of the individual's behavior, then we go about replacing the negative behavior or unwanted behavior by positively rewarding the desired or appropriate replacement behavior— the intention is that over a period of time the acceptable behavior or the behavior that we are looking for will replace the unacceptable behavior because we have positively reinforced the acceptable behavior and ignored or given "if…then" contingences for the negative behavior (see page 96). For example, let's take hitting as a behavior that we want to shape, fade and extinguish. We might say, "*if* you don't hit anyone in the next hour (use a timer) *then* you can use the computer for 15 minutes (use a timer).

Make sure to allow the student to have the positive reinforcement that they earned if they do not hit anyone within the designated hour. We have to be consistent in our delivery of the reinforcer. A good idea is to make a reinforcement inventory listing the reinforcements that will help change the behavior. If a student doesn't care about puzzles, then don't use puzzles as a reinforcement. The reinforcers must be meaningful for the individual.

Primary reinforcers are biological. Food, drink and pleasure are the principal examples of primary reinforcers. We can shape, fade and extinguish behavior the most quickly with primary reinforcers. Secondary reinforcers would be token economies, Lego®, computers, iPads, puzzles and so on.

IMPLEMENTING PBS STRATEGIES: "THE BIG THREE" COMPONENTS

"Catch 'em being good" is a phrase coined by people who use PBS strategies to modify negative or unwanted behavior. The theory is that a reward is given for positive behavior or the behavior that is appropriate and nothing is taken away when negative behavior occurs. We strive to choose a positive reinforcement after positive behavior occurs rather than thinking in terms of punishment following negative behavior. Positive and negative reinforcement can be understood in simple terms as follows: a positive reinforcement is when something good happens after a behavior; negative reinforcement is when something bad happens after a behavior. For example, if you pick up trash on your school yard and put it in the trash bin, then you get a ticket to be used at the school store on Friday (token reward system)—something good happened after the behavior of picking up trash. On the other hand, if you run a red light and a policeman catches you, then you get a ticket, your insurance fees go up and you might even have to attend driver's school. Something bad happened after a behavior or negative reinforcement occurred.

In our fast-paced modern society, we often have a difficult time positively rewarding other people in our daily life or telling others what a great job they have done or how proud we are of their accomplishments. Furthermore, the truth is that societies often have a difficult time with the "idea" of positively rewarding its individuals who have demonstrated "bad" or inappropriate behaviors—a perfect example is the US overcrowded prison system, where punishment is valued over rehabilitation.

Let's take another example: A student hits another peer while getting off the bus. Whether the "behavior" happened immediately prior to school or earlier in the school day, the child may still be being punished three or four hours later for a behavior that occurred in the morning hours. This logic often is that the child should have to endure the PUNISHMENT for their actions for however long the school aide or teacher deems appropriate, and that the punishment matches the inappropriate "behavior." So the child is put in "time out." Let's say that "time out" serves no positive outcome for the individual; rather we are asking a child to sit and do "nothing," or as often times we even hear, you can sit there and "think about what you've done wrong." I believe it is safe to say that no adult would adhere to this ridiculous form of time-wasting agenda and we can rest assured that the child is not sitting in their room thinking about what they did wrong.

The thinking is this, if the child is negatively punished, benched or put in time out for a time "equally equivalent to the inappropriate behavior," then they will certainly remember NOT to do that again! Right? Wrong? Of course, what happens most often is that the child's anger escalates while they are in "time out" and as soon as they return to their desk or activity to work or play on-task, they usually begin to demonstrate inappropriate behavior again. And so it goes on: the adult runs around behind the child, continuously punishing them for their inappropriate behaviors but never understanding the function of the behavior or how the behavior actually served the child while they were doing it in the environment where the behavior occurred. The taking away of stars and earned points on the board in schools, benching at recess and "time out" at school and home, are all punishment strategies that result in continued inappropriate classroom and home behavioral problems. This is because we have succeeded in only temporarily stopping the student doing the behavior rather than working to shape, fade and extinguish it by understanding how the behavior functions for the individual. In other words, was it for attention from an adult or peer? Was it to escape or avoid something in the environment, such as math, language, arts or a task that was too difficult for the individual? Punishment generally serves to escalate inappropriate behavior in an individual who is already angry, and typically leaves a chain of unwanted behaviors in its aftermath.

1. State the rule

State the rule or unwanted behavior. For example, the adult/teacher/parent says, "The rule is no hitting other students in the face." Then we ask the student to repeat the rule by asking them, "What's the rule?" The student repeats, "Don't hit other kids." The student stating the rule afterward allows the student to cognitively "map" the information in the brain. Here comes the important part: immediately after the student verbally states and repeats the rule, reward the student with, "I like the way you are thinking," and/or give them a high five. We want to model the behavior that we are seeking or have asked for, and then REWARD (reinforce) the behavior that the student displays.

2. If…then contingencies

These are "if…then" statements, best stated in the affirmative or what we expect the student to do and what good things will happen when they follow through with what we have asked for in the "rule." Keeping with our student who hit the peer, you say, "*If* you do not hit anyone from now until lunchtime *then* you can have 15 minutes free time on the computer in the afternoon."

We all respond to positive reinforcement, simple case in point. *If* we go to work *then* we get a paycheck. We are being positively rewarded for our good work with a reinforcement or paycheck. Now, if our employer says that due to the state of the economy, we will not be getting paid, then it is highly unlikely that we will return to work the following day. By working hard and getting a paycheck, we are being rewarded for our work well done. It is no different for our children.

Our student doesn't hit for the next three hours, so they get 15 minutes on the computer in the afternoon as promised. More importantly, when the student adheres to the if…then contingency, we cannot assume that the student knows that they have displayed the behavior that we were seeking and then withhold the reward (think of the paycheck analogy). We must give them the reward that we promised in the if…then contingency each time, and immediately after they exhibit the behavior that we were asking of them, until the unacceptable behavior has been extinguished.

What generally falls away from the initial PBS program is the REWARD or reinforcement; then parents, teachers and aides report that the behavior plan (PBS) is not working, when in fact, the reward is missing. We all work for rewards in our life, and without them, we become unmotivated. When we are hungry, we eat. When we go to work, we get a paycheck. *If the student doesn't hit, then they can have computer time.*

3. Two choices

When we redirect, we want to give two choices instead of making the choice for the individual. This allows them to have some measure of power and control over their life. We are not empowered when we are told what to do. For example, "Work on a puzzle" is not empowering, but "Do you want to work on the computer or do a puzzle?" is empowering. Always give the option of "two choices." "You may do the math activity that we are doing or build a house with Lego but you cannot hit, scream and throw objects around the room (tantrum)."

Below is example of how PBS would look using an ABA Antecedent–Behavior–Consequence model:

Antecedent: "Madison sit down please." (A short, simple, not a lot of words, direct verbal prompt—you can even use a full physical gesture with your hand, like a crossing-walk guard or a Maître de in a restaurant to indicate the chair and lead the student to it.)

Behavior: Madison sits down. (Now be careful here: Don't at this point further prompt her to sit up in her chair, put her hands on the table, unfold the napkin, etc. If she sits down, no matter that she is not sitting like a queen, reward her immediately with either a verbal, "I like the way you're sitting Madison," or a tangible reward. I always carry the tangible reward in a baggy or in my pocket so as to continually visually remind the child that there is a REWARD or REINFORCEMENT for complying with a verbal request, be it an on-task activity or an everyday functional skill.)

Consequence: Madison gets a verbal or tangible reward. (Give her a fruit juice gummy bear or say: "I like the way you sat down in the chair. I like the way you're thinking.")

Continuing this behavior as a chained A–B–C model would look like this:

Antecedent: "Now please pick up your fork, Madison."

Behavior: Madison picks up the fork.

Consequence: Madison gets a verbal reward: "I like the way you picked up your fork," and on and on...

Another example:

Behavior: Eating Play-Doh (many of our younger kiddos like to eat objects that are not food).

1. State the RULE clearly:

Adult/teacher: "The rule is no eating the Play-Doh. What's the rule?"

Child: "I can't eat the Play-Doh."

Adult: "I like the way you are thinking, Madison." High five or reinforce her right then. Remember to reinforce the behavior that we are looking for. Our kids are confused as to what the appropriate desired behavior is that is expected from them because they often miss the "natural cues" of the other children in the environment or can't remember or recall what the behavior is that we are expecting or looking for; or it simply may be because of receptive language challenges and they don't know what we are saying or asking of them.

2. Give "If...then" contingencies:

If you don't eat Play-Doh for the next _____ (fill in the blank e.g. 1 hour (?), 15 minutes (?) from now until lunch) then you can have _____ (e.g. computer time, be my assistant, pass out the paints etc.). In this way, the child is rewarded for NOT eating the Play-Doh instead of being punished in time out (where they do nothing, are humiliated and begin to get angry so the situation escalates).

We might even take the opportunity to say, "You know I like the way that you are NOT eating Play-Doh," right after we give the "if...then" contingency (that way we are certain that the child knows what we are looking for—for them NOT to eat the Play-Doh). Reinforce the behavior that we are looking for!

3. Now we redirect with two choices:

"You have two choices, you can pick another activity—either _____ (painting, drawing, Lego, etc.) or _____ (book, puzzle, books on CD, etc.). What do you want to do?"

The child picks one of the activities and goes to it. (If the child does not pick an activity from the two choices, then you can say; "Let me help you; you picked books on CD," and use a physical gesture (i.e. help the child up and over to the books on CD center). Either way (whether you made the choice or they made the choice), REINFORCE THEIR CHOICE because this is the behavior that we are looking for. Say, "I like the way that you picked books on CD and that you are not eating Play-Doh! I like the way that you are thinking."

Reinforcement is the KEY! The BIG THREE will help us to shape, fade and eventually extinguish unwanted behavior. The important thing to remember is that the classroom, community and home environment don't have to be "battle grounds." It's easy, just remember to say, "I like the way you're thinking!"

CHAPTER 5

Social Ability: You Dance and So Shall I

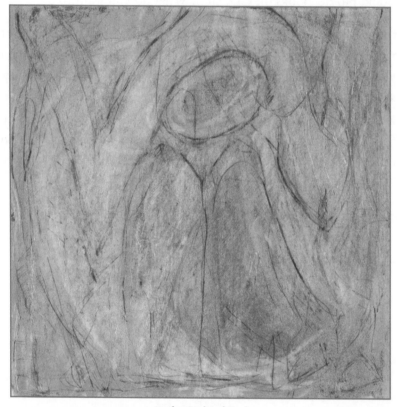

Art by Gerhard Beck

"If someone doesn't want to come out of their shell and talk to me, I'll just find another shell."

JULIAN ARSI, 13 YEARS OLD

We need to be teaching the fundamental social skills of my turn, your turn, initiating and taking turns in taking turns in simple dialogue and so much more. Our kids, because of the lack of a facilitated role-playing modeling of social skills, are growing up and transitioning out of the school system with a very splintered social skills set. This splintered skill set is not preparing them for the workplace or inclusion in their community. What if the government mandated a curriculum that aligned itself with academic standards that specifically addressed social skills, and was facilitated by the teacher and teaching assistants in the classroom, for both students with disabilities and NT students? This social skills curriculum would include teaching social skills sets in an inclusive setting, starting in pre-kindergaten with text and formal lessons, and would align itself with the curriculum and go all the way up to middle school.

Arnold Miller, who pioneered the Cognitive–Developmental Systems Approach for Children on the Autism Spectrum, breaks down autism into two types of autistic children: those with closed system disorders and those with system-forming disorders. "Scattered" children with system-forming disorders require organized, highly structured settings in order to help them organize their functioning and to experience the world in predictable terms. Children with closed systems may initially need order but then require the challenge that disorder introduces (Miller and Chretien 2007, p.32).

Social skills deficits are criteria for the eligibility of autism. The DSM-5 (Diagnostic and Statistical Manual of Mental Disorders, 5th edition) explains social skills challenges in individuals with autism as persistent difficulties in the social use of verbal and nonverbal communications as manifested by all of the following:

1. Deficits in using communication for social purposes, such as greeting and sharing information, in a manner that is appropriate for social context.

2. Impairment in the ability to change communication to match context of the needs of the listener, such as speaking differently in a classroom than on a playground, talking differently to a child than to an adult, and avoiding use of overly formal language.

3. Difficulties following rules for conversation and storytelling, such as taking turns in conversation, rephrasing when misunderstood, and knowing how to use verbal and nonverbal signals to regulate interaction.

4. Difficulties understanding what is not explicitly stated (e.g. making inferences) and nonliteral or ambiguous meaning of language (e.g. idioms, humor, metaphors, multiple meanings that depend on the context for interpretation).

5. The deficits result in functional limitations in effective communication, social participation, social relationships, academic achievement, or occupational performance, individually or in combination.

6. The onset of symptoms is in the early developmental period (but deficits may not become fully manifest until social communication demands exceed limited capacities).

7. The symptoms are not attributable to another medical or neurological condition or to low abilities in the domains of word structure and grammar, and are not better explained by autism spectrum disorder, intellectual disability (intellectual developmental disorder), global developmental delay, or another mental disorder.

(APA 2013)

A COLD, HARD FACT

Throughout an autistic child's life, support from an active team of parents, teachers, peers and other professionals is required to teach essential and functional life skills. For the purposes of clarity, we are defining functional life skills as the necessary skills and tasks that contribute to the successful, independent functioning of an individual in adulthood. The ability to plan, organize and take care of such things as cooking, cleaning, shopping, dressing, personal hygiene, medical and dental care, money management, etc. are essential skills necessary to help a child reach their highest potential into adulthood.

Life skills are vital and important markers for future success and independence, and yet people will not dismiss a person because they cannot cook or clean. An individual can be supported to manage money, make a doctor's appointment or go to the grocery store. If they can't hold down a job, or go to college, there are many things they can do to give meaning to their life. But without the ability to connect with others, meaningful social connections outside of family members or paid staff will be difficult, if not non-existent.

Social connections are an intrinsic part of who we are as humans. Social connection is critical to our very beings, and core social skills—or lack of them—will determine how included or segregated a child/adult will be within the family unit, the community, in a job or career, and in building meaningful friendships throughout their lifetime. This is not to say that people cannot be loved—and love—without social skills. Of course they can. We love our children, our brothers, sisters and others with autism, even when they lack social skills—but will others? Will society pause long enough to care about them?

IN THE BEGINNING THERE WAS IMPAIRED SOCIAL UNDERSTANDING…

Without the ability to empathize and understand other people's emotions, feelings, needs and ideas, kids will become isolated adults. For kids with severe autism, the focus on self, or "Mindblindness," often appears to completely exclude other people's feelings and needs—so we must find a way to help them to connect with others (Baron-Cohen 1999).

Autistic kids need intense, repetitive modeling of goal-oriented social skills in order to use these skills naturally in everyday situations. As we have previously discussed, movement and music—and other forms of art—offer a creative, non-threatening, structured forum to target social deficits and practice social skills.

When kids first join an Autism Movement Therapy® session, we see a common trajectory in their reactions, behavior and evolution in the groups. Initial participation in the groups often reveals some, if not most, of the following challenges in the first few group sessions:

- Sensory overload (including lights, sounds, proximity to group).

- Fear/discomfort with "newness" of group, environment and/or facilitator.

- Separation from parents (anxiety).

- Difficulty understanding requests/directions of facilitator; communication deficits.

- Lack of focus; difficulty joining group.

- Difficulty staying on task.

- Inability to follow or understand routines.

- Challenges in gross and fine body movements.

- Inability to relate to and work with others in the group.

- Inability to use imagination in opening/closing circles and in creative movements.

- Challenges in letting loose and having natural play/fun.

PRIORITIZE THE MOST CRITICAL CHALLENGES IN ORDER OF IMPORTANCE TO SUCCESS

From the very first AMT session, the challenges listed—and others you might experience as a parent with your child—can be addressed best by identifying which ones are most disruptive to your child's everyday life. For example, what causes the most disruptive or aggressive behaviors in your child? What difficulties impair school performance the most? What area of delay or impairment causes the most disruption in the home or community?

It can be assumed that whatever challenges are most apparent in initial AMT sessions are also typical of how a child will react in most other new environments. Though your child may display many of the challenges listed above, if the most difficult challenge is, for example, sensory overload in the environment, it's likely that they experience the same problem when entering other new environments. In this example, sensory overload would become your primary (first) target in an AMT session, because without diminishing sensory overload other learning cannot take place.

Here is an example of this issue written as goal, objective, outcome and process steps:

Goal: Reduce sensory overload in new environments.

Objective: The child will learn new strategies to help calm/regulate self in new environments.

Outcome: The child will be able to adapt more easily to new environments, using self-calming techniques and strategies.

Process steps:

1. Discuss the new environment and what might occur.

2. Visit the new environment in advance of participation, if necessary or helpful.

3. Provide visuals. Show pictures of the new environment, the facilitator, or even a (generic) photo of kids dancing. We use YouTube a lot to look up new ideas, places and things to support discussions about new and scary places, for example. This is an excellent tool for all skills across the board.

4. Practice calming techniques before starting an AMT session (breathing, walking, stretching, having a drink of water, etc.).

5. Listen to the recommended AMT music with your child before sessions (priming).

6. When entering the new environment, help your child to determine safety to approach other children.

7. On arrival, give a verbal greeting ("hello") or non-verbal greeting (high five, thumbs up, etc.).

Definition: When kids are aware of what to expect, their anxieties and fear can be reduced. Seeing a photo or video examples of the aforementioned steps can help to prepare them for new environments. Practice, role playing and pretending help to train the brain for new situations or that something new is going to happen.

Rationale: Diminishing sensory overload helps kids to deal with everyday transitions in new environments, and opens up pathways to other learning. When sensory overload occurs, think of this as a blockage in your sink: things (learning) cannot get through until the drain is clear.

When/where/comments

- Describe or brainstorm the times when your child was successful in a new environment and how it felt to overcome the fear or anxiety.

- Discuss and practice meeting new people.

- Discuss how to decide if a new environment is safe.

- Discuss how music and movement helps our bodies to relax and calm.

- Discuss good listening skills and how we learn new things by "putting on our good listening ears."

- Discuss previous successes and benefits discovered in new environments in the past.

- Discuss and reinforce how to introduce ourselves to others.

Model/role play at home

- Stand in front of a mirror with your child. Move body parts and ask your child to look in the mirror and follow your movements.

- Ask your child to show you how different animals might move or sound. "A rabbit hops." "An elephant might sound like this…"

- Have other family members/friends join in the fun. Line everybody up (place a taped dot on the floor) and move across the floor, one person at a time. Reinforce turn taking.

- Practice sitting criss-cross applesauce. Clap hands to syllables of your name as you say it ("My name is Sho-sha-na"); have your child model your actions saying their name as they clap to the syllables.

- Practice (model) different types of verbal and non-verbal greetings.

For some, we see that after just one AMT session the initial fears or challenges of joining a new group, including the sounds and new people, etc., "softens" the edges and makes room for an instantly positive experience. For most, there is an eagerness to come again and enjoy the ongoing classes. Yet for others, the process takes more time.

BOX 5.1 USE ROLE PLAYING FOR SKILL BUILDING

Your car is an excellent place to work on role play and rehearsing skills. Turn the radio off; take headsets and ear buds off! Actively engage with your child. Ask your child what they think and feel. Talk about what is experienced in the AMT environment. Talk about all the skills you want to encourage. Remember, repeating and replaying various scenarios is most helpful in learning and retaining new skills.

AMT PREDICTABILITY HELPS GROW CONFIDENCE

In Chapter 3 we discussed the pattern and sequencing of musical notes and patterns. The patterns we hear, that we use our body parts to create, and even the vibrations we feel in our bodies (auditory, vestibular, sensory, etc.), set the stage for following a "road map" of AMT sequencing. This road map, being predictable, strengthens brain connectivity and helps wake up the brain to support kids to follow routines, learn to improvise and use their imaginations. These developments and the continued practice of these skills outside of the AMT setting will have a direct and significant impact on learning new social skills.

Sometimes, in trying to improve social skills, simple strategies are overlooked. How we gain confidence and understanding by interacting with others is taken for granted at times. For example, a child who is put in a special day class misses out on the opportunity to model NT peers in the general education setting. A child who does not participate in community sports, arts, music and other activities because they might have a meltdown (or other reasons—fill in the blank…), will miss out on very important life lessons.

When we process most of the activities of an average day for our child (picking up their clothes, choosing their clothes for them, brushing their teeth or hair, getting their mail from the mail box, etc., etc.) we are blocking their road to knowledge and skill building. Ultimately, this has a direct impact on social skills. After all, if we expect little from our children, they will likely produce little for themselves. In doing "things" for our kids, instead of allowing them to have a go themselves (even if it is not perfect), we do not allow them to build the self-esteem, confidence and self-determination that will serve them in the future. When our efforts make their life "easier," they learn little about self-sufficiency, diligence, and working with others. They are more likely to "atrophy" in social awareness and connectivity skills.

We cannot emphasize enough the importance of treating your child with autism as you would treat any other child in terms of pushing for excellence in self-management and care. It is important for us to find the courage to believe in our children—even when what we see often leads us to believe that they cannot learn. As parents, many of us feel pangs of fear and guilt. We want to protect our child at every turn. But is this practical? Not in the real world. We need to balance protection and support with—as we've said before—raising the bar. Believe in your child's possibilities, not their limitations, and great things will happen at their own, individual level of accomplishment.

Sad, but true: One day you won't be here to take care of your child. One day they will need to rely on themselves and, likely, others for their care. That is the inevitable truth. The more they can do for themselves and connect with others, the less you will have to worry about their future care, safety and happiness.

BOX 5.2 INCLUSION WHENEVER, WHEREVER POSSIBLE

Inclusion supports social awareness and skill building. If children are not exposed to different everyday environments to grow skills, connection to the real world is limited. AMT encourages siblings and typical peers to join in. All domains of the arts, whether music, movement, fine art, drama, theater and other creative expressions are perfect for using in an inclusion model. If you are considering starting an AMT program in your area, it is always good to invite NT individuals to join in. AMT is a highly effective tool in bringing everyone together to have fun and grow skills for all.

ARC in Herkimer, New York, uses AMT as an adult social skills weekly program, with refreshments served afterwards to encourage friendships.

AMT STUDENTS SHOW TREMENDOUS GROWTH

The following are ways in which AMT helps our students:

- Supports adaptation to new surroundings, people and the instructor.

- Supports adaptation to loud noises, music and laughter.

- Lowers social and general anxiety.

- Provides understanding starting point (the dot) to generalize in everyday skill building.

- Adds excitement (in the home environment) by getting ready for, and going to, sessions.

- Builds upon ability to follow routines and other structured activities.

- Develops ability to remain on task.

- Promotes active interaction and engagement with other students and instructor.

- Reinforces and teaches the expectation of turn taking (my turn, your turn).

- Supports active participation in opening circle; use of language, communication and imagination.

- Grows and encourages empathy toward others.

- Grows ability and desire to lead when offered opportunities to do so.

- Grows ability and desire to follow others.

- Develops compliance and follow-through.

- Has direct impact on self-determination and self-direction.

- NT siblings and peers are supported to embrace and understand differences, and to become good role models for all.

Over time, these improvements—individually and collectively—demonstrate a greater ability to generalize multiple skills across other environments. When children generalize social skills in a creative, relaxed and supportive environment, those skills are more easily adapted to everyday situations.

Such has been the case with Shoshana, who comes to AMT classes on a regular basis. She tells us she "loves the music, the exercise, and Ms. Lara." Years ago, when Shoshana first started AMT classes, she presented with many of the challenges previously listed. Over time, her ability to lead class exercises and to improvise has improved greatly. She is an alert and active participant in the normal routines of the group. Her self-esteem and awareness of others in the group is superior. In the AMT environment, we do not see the anxiety Shoshana sometimes demonstrates in other environments. AMT is a place where Shoshana feels safe and flourishes, and, she is always ready to stand on her dot to begin the class.

RELATING TO OTHERS IN CLASS AND SOCIAL SITUATIONS

On the following page are a few more examples of goals, objectives, outcomes and process steps used in AMT sessions to develop and support understanding of routines, movements and expectations. *Note: The "dot" used in the first example can (and should) be used outside of AMT sessions to generalize everyday life and social lessons. A good question to ask the child is "Where is your dot/starting place?"*

You are encouraged to use this format to create your own vision for your child's or students' other areas of need, putting those things down in writing as a plan.

Goal: Improve simple social skill of greeting others.

Objective: The child will acknowledge others in class with appropriate greetings.

Outcome: The child will begin to use simple greetings without a verbal prompt.

Process steps:

1. Stop and look to see who is in the class.

2. Determine safety to approach other children.

3. Give verbal greeting ("hello") or non-verbal greeting (high five, thumbs up, etc.).

Definition: When kids are aware of and acknowledge the presence of others, they can let others know they are interested in connecting with and joining them in the group setting.

Rationale: Growing appropriate basic social skills helps kids to relate to others and improves social awareness/self-esteem. Social awareness supports inclusion and acceptance while building connectivity. When kids look outwards to acknowledge others around them, they are more likely to be included, be able to empathize, and feel they are part of a group.

When/where/comments

- Describe or brainstorm the times when children would need this skill (in class, new situations, in the classroom, after-school care, camp and when meeting new people).

- Discuss stranger danger/safety in general terms to outline when it is appropriate to greet new people.

- Discuss how to decide if a person is safe, including learning to interpret body language, age, mannerisms and different environments.

- Discuss different ways to greet people—verbal and non-verbal.

- Discuss and reinforce how to introduce ourselves to others; model different greetings.

- Discuss various places/situations where the child might not know people who greet them (e.g. grocery store, the park, etc.).

Model/role play

Greetings that your child has practiced in AMT classes (i.e., "Hi, my name is Shoshana. Can I play with you?" or "My name is Emma. What's your name?") can be generalized for every day situations. Give your child various role play scenarios such as:

- You go to the park and want to join in play with others.

- You want to join the kids playing a game on the school yard.

- You move to a new school.

- You join a new social skills group.

- You go to your church or synagogue.

- You join a baseball, soccer or football team.

- You are invited to a birthday party.

- You are going to a relative's house.

- You want to join the kids playing next door/across the street.

Desired Outcomes

On the following page is a list of outcomes in areas that, over a period of time, we should see progress. Remember to meet the student where they are at any given point in time. Meeting the marks and continually raising the bar of expectation is the hallmark of AMT.

- Practice having a family member or friend knock on your front door and have your child greet them. Teach stranger danger awareness in these lessons. When is it safe or not safe to open the door?

- Have your child practice greetings in all everyday environments (e.g. the grocery store, bank, doctor's office). To grow this skill even further (or raise the bar), give your child the money to hand to the cashier and use words to say, "Here is the money." Have your child check in at the dentist's office: "Hi, I'm Jane. I am here for my appointment." At the bank, demonstrate filling out a deposit slip (if possible) and then greet the teller… "Hello." Or, "We are here to make a deposit."

- Use everyday environments daily! We miss all kinds of opportunities to have our children process social steps. We tend to be in a rush and without a second thought we just do the task at hand ourselves. Slow down. Prompt your child to do everyday (grown-up) tasks for themselves in addition to greeting others.

- Set up pretend scenarios at home where your child takes a turn being the one to serve someone else, open the door or answer the phone.

- Have your child read to you (or read to them if they cannot read) lots and lots of books on being a good friend.

STANDING ON THE DOT: A PLACE TO START

In AMT classes, the dot is real. In life, the dot can come to symbolize a starting place for other things. The dot—actual or metaphorical can become a prompt to "wake up the brain" to process action steps (e.g. "Where is your dot? Where do we (you) start so we can solve this problem?") Discuss the "dot" in a way that helps kids to generalize everyday tasks (i.e. If you have a place to start—the "dot," real or imaginary—can help you to clear your mind to see the next steps).

Goal: Learn to stand on the dot as a starting point.

Objective: The student will learn to take their place on the dot as their starting point in the class, first with a verbal prompt and eventually without a prompt.

Outcome: The real and/or metaphorical dot will serve as a prompt to improve active listening, focus and follow-through on directions given or in daily life tasks.

Process steps:

1. "Wake up the brain"; listen and watch for a verbal or nonverbal cue/request (i.e. stand on the dot).

2. Observe and watch other group members taking up position on their dot to start the session.

3. Walk to, and stand in place on the dot (model if necessary); wait for instructions for the movement to start.

4. Begin movement when the facilitator directs.

Definition: Standing on the dot helps the student to understand where to position their body (and mind) in order to start the routines/lessons.

Rationale: A person needs to know where they need to be to begin a process step for everyday tasks and needs. (In this case, to begin the movements?)

Where/when/how comments

- How do I begin to process/start a given process or step?

- If I have a specific place to start, I can use that (dot) as a way to wake up my brain to take on the next step/process.

- When I can focus on a starting point (in this case the dot,) it can allow for and support the next step (directions and movement) to make better sense.

- How can use of the "dot" be generalized and used in other ways to process other skills in my life?

Model/role play with feedback

- Students will learn to automatically move to and stand on their dot to start the session.

- Use video modeling (see below). As parents, you can create a baseline (present level of performance) by filming your child to show them where they are at. Continue to video progress/improvement to show growth and achievements. "Show them," don't "tell them." With positive reinforcement, kids can see themselves, which really helps them relate to self and supports their personal awareness and self-esteem. Use questions such as "What do you see?" or "Are you following the group?"

- Parents/professionals can use the dot to generalize everyday process steps. "Okay, at this point, we take a breath, focus and work on the next step to figure out what comes next."

VIDEO MODELING: SHOW ME, DON'T TELL ME

We need to help kids with autism "see" themselves in a way that helps them to understand and relate to the world around them. A child might not understand what we tell them, but can relate more easily to what we show them. This is true for most people. In better understanding our behaviors and how they impact others, we can make better choices about how we act and behave.

It's difficult enough for most people to improve or change behaviors they do not see, understand or necessarily even appear to care about. But it's especially hard to relate to self when you are autistic. We all need to have awareness, and some understanding of our behaviors in relationship to people, places and things around us in order to build social skills. Showing, not telling, is an active and positive way to let our children see, learn and grow.

We have used the following methods to support visual video modeling:

- Film children behaving in the desired way for discussion later.

- Use online sources such as YouTube to show everyday situations and positive behavior.

- Use an educational source we like called "Video Modeling and Video Self-Modeling."[1]

- Have your child film others practicing desired behavior—let them view the world and social skills from the other side of the camera.

Filming children behaving in a desirable way for discussion later

When we use positive reinforcement as our guiding principle, good choices and behaviors can be modeled by filming children when they are practicing desired behaviors. This can be film in real-life circumstances, or film in role playing.

Ideas for role playing might include: how to answer the door; using an automated teller machine at the bank; engaging in play at a park. Use your imagination. Use everyday situations to make video diaries of appropriate social skills.

We work with our AMT student Emma outside of AMT classes on everyday social and academic skills. Recently, Emma turned 13 and wanted to begin to take on more responsibilities as a teenager yet, (as one example) she was extremely nervous about ordering food at her favorite take-out place. We role-rehearsed extensively in advance, and then turned the camera on her at the counter ordering food. Later, we viewed the footage with her so she could see where she excelled and where she might improve in the future. She is now ordering her food more happily and confidently and reports: "It really helped me to watch myself ordering my burrito. It made me feel good to do that."

After you have filmed your child in a particular setting, use the footage over several different periods of time (days, weeks or months) to reinforce the values filmed. Seeing themselves in positive interactions helps kids feel good about themselves—and we all want to feel good about ourselves, right?

Note: we do not suggest filming your child during periods of undesired behaviors, meltdowns or other inappropriate activity. We want to reinforce positive behaviors and PBS and not focus on undesired behaviors or activities.

---

1   Available at www.vsmproject.pbworks.com/w/page/27900729/Samples.

Using online sources for video-modeling

YouTube can be a useful tool to show everyday situations and positive behavior.

We used video modeling again with Emma in relation to helping her overcome her extreme fear of birds. Though she still fears birds, her loud screams and shaking have diminished significantly by using YouTube videos as a tool. In this case, while sitting with Emma, we chose appropriate videos about sea gulls. We looked up "sea gulls on the beach" and "sea gulls flying in flocks," and found "I'm a Silly Sea Gull, Sing-Along for Kids" (Reid 2009). Soon after reviewing videos (on different days, repeating the exercise), Emma painted a sea gull, denoting a closer connection to accepting the birds. "I feel a little better about birds now," she reports.

Nearly any situation or place or scenario can be looked up somewhere on the internet as a tool for modeling. Just be sure to monitor what is watched, so that appropriate content can be viewed at your discretion.

Have your child film other people, places and things

Let your child view the world and social skills from the other side of the camera. This is an excellent way to grow a variety of skills. Autism by its very nature is a self-centered condition. If we redirect self to others, we are opening up a door to many social and other skills. Empathy, understanding and perspective taking are among the most important. Putting a camera in your kid's hands also promotes artistic vision, creativity and learning. At first things might be out of focus or may not make sense to your child's eye. That is part of the process! Over time, we often see kids actively getting into the subject matter and the perspective of the world around them. How they see the world is an excellent opportunity for family dialogue, family projects and who knows, maybe even a future in photography or film production?

LET'S REVIEW THE BASIC CHARACTERISTICS OF SOCIAL SKILLS

The values and skills necessary for basic skills building include the following characteristics:

- Skills are goal-directed and oriented (they have a functional purpose).

- Skills and behaviors may require a person to use more than one skill or behavior at the same time for the same goal.

- Different social skills might/will be used in different situations (e.g. at a job vs. personal communications).

- Social skills can be taught, demonstrated, modeled, practiced and learned.

- Different social skills are used at different times and in many different contexts (e.g. a child needs to be taught about no talking to a stranger vs. meeting a new person).

In Temple Grandin and Sean Barron's book, *The Unwritten Rules of Social Relationships* (Grandin and Barron 2005), the authors worked together to create "The 10 Unwritten Rules of Social Relationships." These include:

1. Rules are not absolute. They are situation-based and people-based.

2. Not everything is equally important in the grand scheme of things.

3. Everyone in the world makes mistakes. It doesn't have to ruin your day.

4. Honesty is different than diplomacy.

5. Being polite is appropriate in any situation.

6. Not everyone who is nice to me is my friend.

7. People act differently in public than they do in private.

8. Know when you're turning people off.

9. "Fitting in" is often tied to looking and sounding like you fit in.

10. People are responsible for their own behaviors.

NOW GO OUT AND MAKE IT HAPPEN!

There is clearly so much more to teaching and learning social skills than we have explored in this chapter. In fact, learning basic and functional social skills can take a lifetime for some and could fill libraries on concepts of the how, when, where, why and what of developing social skills. Our point in addressing the basics in this book is to show how AMT is interrelated and connected to building social skills through arts, imagination and process.

The successes we have seen and enjoyed in the kiddos we've worked with over years of AMT classes, camps and private clients, and in using the arts in general, are connected to the esteem and joy we feel in having witnessed those successes and to having been a part of them.

We now encourage you to take what you have learned in this book and go out into your kid's world to implement, practice and play with the suggested strategies and see what happens. We have no doubt you will experience transformations beyond your wildest imaginations over time, and that these strategies will simply become a way of life and living with your child, your students and autism.

IN CONCLUSION

It's a big world out there, ever growing, ever changing. Let's make sure that we are preparing our kids with autism to meet that world head on. It's no longer good enough to have our youth merely learn to read and write and graduate from a public school setting. They need a whole new group of skill sets to maneuver their way in the workplace and community. Just like we help the children find their position on the dance floor using painter's tape, so we must provide them with the skills and tools to be successful and take their place in the world. Parents must stop only living in hope and begin to ask for a "seat at the table," for their sons and daughters.

Transitioning from the school setting to either a college, a job or a day center program, and how our young adults with autism will do that, is directly related to the skills that we make certain they have access to. A strong music and movement program, and the arts, assist with developing the higher-level thinking skills necessary to help establish a strong foundational roadmap for life.

So once again we honor Louise Kavadlo and her words "If I had had this available to me when I was younger, I wouldn't be the person that I am today." What Louise means is that at the age of 67 she thinks she would not have had as many challenges as she continues to have to this day had she had access to AMT when she was growing up. Since the writing of this book, Louise has assisted me for an Autism Movement Therapy certification workshop at Marymount Manhattan College in New York City. Not long after the February workshop I received a beautiful card from Louise in the mail. She had made the card herself—a lovely "thank you" card with a carefully made flower of pink, green and purple construction paper, laid out on the thick card stock with such care and attention to detail. Inside Louise wrote:

February 23, 2015

Dear Joanne,

Thank you so much for the check ($100.00) and having me as your Assistant. I have Asperger's Syndrome; my sister Joan doesn't. Dance is healthy from infancy to the Geriatric set. Let's all Dance to Life, Peace, Joy!

Louise Kavadlo

Let's pledge to provide access to the arts to every child, so that they can reach their full potential and take their rightful "seat at the table."

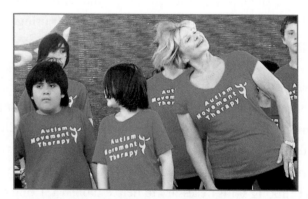

World Special Olympics 2015, Los Angeles, CA
Photo by Diane Bernstein

References

Baron-Cohen, S. (1999) *Mindblindness: An Essay on Autism and Theory of Mind*. Cambridge, MA: MIT Press.

Begley, S. (2007) *Train Your Mind, Change Your Brain*. London: Constable.

Chan, J. M. and O'Reilly, M. F. (2008) "A Social Stories™ intervention package for students with autism in inclusive classroom settings." *Journal of Applied Behavior Analysis 41*, 3, 405–409.

Cohn, A. M. (2001) "Positive behavioral Supports: Information for Educators." *National Association of School Psychologists*. Available at www.nasponline.org/resources/factsheets/pbs_fs.aspx, accessed on 18 August 2015.

Doidge, N. (2007) *The Brain that Changes Itself: Stories of Personal Triumph from the Frontiers of Brain Science*. New York, NY: Penguin.

Durand, V. M. and Crimmins, D. B. (1992) *The Motivation Assessment Scale (MAS) Administration Guide*. Topeka, KS: Monaco and Associates.

Durand, V. M. and Merges, E. (2001) "Functional communication training: A contemporary behavior analytic intervention for problem behaviors." *Focus on Autism and Other Developmental Disabilities 16*, 2, 110–119.

Ellis, N. C. (1996) "Working memory in the acquisition of vocabulary and syntax: putting language in good order." *The Quarterly Journal of Experimental Psychology: Section A 49*,1, 234–250.

Frazier, T. W., Keshavan, M. S., Minshew, N. J. and Hardan, A. Y. (2012) "A two-year longitudinal MRI study of the corpus callosum in autism." *Journal of Autism and Developmental Disorders 42*, 11, 2312–2322.

Grandin, T. (2013) *The Autistic Brain: Helping Different Kinds of Minds Succeed*. Boston, MA: Houghton Mifflin Harcourt.

Grandin, T. and Barron, S. (2005) *The Unwritten Rules of Social Relationships*. Fort Worth, TX: Future Horizons.

Hartshorn, K., Olds, L., Field, T., Delage, J., Cullen, C. and Escalona, A. (2001) "Creative movement therapy benefits children with autism." *Early Child Development and Care 166*,1, 1–5.

Kapp, S. K. (2013) "Empathizing with sensory and movement differences: Moving toward sensitive understanding of autism." *Frontiers in Integrative Neuroscience 38*. Doi 10.3389/fnint.2013.00038.

Kranowitz, C. S. (2005) *The Out-of-Sync Child: Recognizing and Coping with Sensory Processing Disorder*. New York, NY: Perigee.

Landau, E. (2012) "Music: It's in your head, changing your brain." *CNN*. Available at www.cnn.com/2012/05/26/health/mental-health/music-brain-science, accessed on 16 May 2015.

Lara, J. (2009) "Autism Movement Therapy®: *aut-erobics®* movement and music sensory integration to 'wake up the brain'." *Autism/Asperger's Digest*, February/March, 39–40.

Lord, C., Rutter, M., Goode, S., Heemsbergen, J., Jordan, H., Mawhood, L. and Schopler, E. (1989) "Autism diagnostic observation schedule: A standardized observation of communicative and social behavior." *Journal of Autism and Developmental Disorders 19*, 2, 185–212.

Mahadevan, S. (2015) "Albert Einstein's great passion for music." Available at www.shankarmahadevacademy.com/community/articles/view/2/, accessed on 16 May 2015.

Men, W., Falk, D., Sun, T., Chen, W., *et al.* (2013) "The corpus callosum of Albert Einstein's brain: another clue to his high intelligence?" *Brain: A Journal of Neurology.* doi:10.1093/brain/awt252.

Miller, A. and Chretien, K. (2007) *The Miller Method: Developing the Capacities of Children on the Autism Spectrum.* London: Jessica Kingsley Publishers.

McGarry, L. M. and Russo, F. A. (2011) "Mirroring in dance/movement therapy: Potential mechanisms behind empathy enhancement." *The Arts in Psychotherapy 38*, 3, 178–184.

Reid, R. (2009) *Children's Jukebox, Second Edition: The Select Subject Guide to Children's Musical Recordings.* Washington, DC: ALA Publishers.

Rutter, M., Le Couteur, A. and Lord, C. (2005) *Autism Diagnostic Interview-Revised.* Los Angeles, CA: Western Psychological Services.

Sacks, O. (2007) *Musicophilia: Tales of Music and the Brain.* New York, NY: Alfred A. Knopf.

Schopler, E., Reichler, R. J., DeVellis, R. F. and Daly, K. (1980) "Toward objective classification of childhood autism: Childhood Autism Rating Scale (CARS)." *Journal of Autism and Developmental Disorders 10*, 1, 91–103.

Shore, S. M. (2002) *Beyond the Wall: Personal Experiences with Autism and Asperger Syndrome.* Shawnee Mission, KS: Autism Asperger Publishing Co.

Shore, S. M. (2014) Teaching music to and experiencing sensory issues. Insights for teaching children with autism. [PowerPoint presentation]

Stewart, L., von Kriegstein, K., Warren, J. D. and Griffiths, T. D. (2006) "Music and the brain: disorders of musical listening." *Brain 129*, 10, 2533–2553.

Torres, E. B. and Donnellan, A. M. (2015) "Editorial for research topic 'Autism: The Movement Perspective'." *Frontiers in Integrative Neuroscience 9*, 12. Doi 10.3389/fnint.2015.00012.

Toth, K., Munson, J., Meltzoff, A. N.and Dawson, G. (2006) "Early predictors of communication development in young children with autism spectrum disorder: Joint attention, imitation, and toy play." *Journal of Autism and Developmental Disorders 36*, 8, 993–1005.

Wang, K. (2014) "The importance of art in special education." Available at www.friendshipcircle. org/blog/2014/04/03/the-importance-of-the-arts-in-special-education/, accessed on 12 June 2015.

Woo, C. C. and Leon, M. (2013) "Environmental enrichment as an effective treatment for autism: a randomized controlled trial." *Behavioral Neuroscience 127*, 4, 487–497.

Index